MANUAL OF
ACUTE CORONARY CARE

JOIN US ON THE INTERNET VIA WWW, GOPHER, FTP OR EMAIL:

WWW: http://www.thomson.com
GOPHER: gopher.thomson.com
FTP: ftp.thomson.com
EMAIL: findit@kiosk.thomson.com

A service of I(T)P®

MANUAL OF
ACUTE CORONARY CARE

A GUIDE TO PATIENT MANAGEMENT

Editors

Michael Walsh, MD, FRCPI, FESC
Raymond Meleady, MB, MRCPI
Shahid Junejo, MB, BS, MRCPI
Ian Graham, FRCPI, FCCP
Gerard Gearty, ScD(TCD), FRCPI

ALTMAN
An Imprint of Chapman & Hall

London · Weinheim · New York · Tokyo · Melbourne · Madras

Chapman & Hall, 2–6 Boundary Row, London SE1 8HN, UK

Chapman & Hall, 2–6 Boundary Row, London SE1 8HN, UK

Chapman & Hall GmbH, Pappelallee 3, 69469 Weinheim, Germany

Chapman & Hall USA, 115 Fifth Avenue, New York, NY 10003, USA

Chapman & Hall Japan, ITP-Japan, Kyowa Building, 3F, 2-2-1 Hirakawacho, Chiyoda-ku, Tokyo 102, Japan

Chapman & Hall Australia, 102 Dodds Street, South Melbourne, Victoria 3205, Australia

Chapman & Hall India, R. Seshadri, 32 Second Main Road, CIT East, Madras 600 035, India

First edition 1998

© 1998 Chapman and Hall

Original released as *Acute Coronary Care*, by the Irish Heart Foundation, 1993

Typeset in 10/12 Janson by Pure Tech India Ltd, Pondicherry

Printed in Britain at the Alden Press Ltd

ISBN 0 1860360114 (PB)

A catalogue record for this book is available from the British Library

Library of Congress Catalog Card Number: 97–69684

∞ Printed on acid-free text paper, manufactured in accordance with ANSI/NISO Z39.48-1992 (Permanence of Paper).

CONTENTS

List of contributors   vii
Preface to the second edition   ix
Preface to the first edition   xi
Acknowledgements   xiii
List of abbreviations   xv

 1. General guidelines   1
 2. Management of myocardial infarction in the CCU   21
 3. Right ventricular infarction   23
 4. Post-myocardial infarction angina   25
 5. Lipids – post-myocardial infarction management   27
 6. Follow up treatment post-myocardial infarction   29
 7. Complications of myocardial infarction   31
 8. Interventions   59
 9. Investigations post-myocardial infarction   63
10. Cardiac rehabilitation and secondary prevention   65

Appendices
    A. COMMONLY USED DRUGS   69
    B. CARDIOPULMONARY RESUSCITATION
       PROTOCOLS   79
    C. AMERICAN HEART ASSOCIATION GUIDELINES
       ON TEMPORARY PACING   83
    D. INTERESTING ECGS   85
    E. CORONARY RISK CHART   91
    F. USEFUL REFERENCES AND SUGGESTED
       READING   95
Index   97

CONTRIBUTORS

Peter Crean, MSc, FRCPI, Consultant Cardiologist, St James's Hospital, Dublin.

Binayak Deb, MRCP, DipCard (London), Consultant Cardiologist, Bombay, India.

Gerard Gearty, ScD(TCD), FRCPI, formerly Consultant Cardiologist, St James's Hospital, Dublin; Lecturer in Postgraduate Cardiology at Royal City of Dublin Hospital.

Ian Graham, FRCPI, FCCP, Consultant Cardiologist, Adelaide and Meath Hospitals; Professor of Epidemiology and Preventive Medicine, Royal College of Surgeons in Ireland, Dublin.

Shahid Junejo, MB, BS, MRCPI, Registrar in Clinical Cardiology, St James's Hospital, Dublin.

Raymond Meleady, MB, MRCPI, Research Fellow in Cardiology, Adelaide Hospital, Dublin.

Michael Walsh, MD, FRCPI, FESC, Head of Department, Department of Cardiology, St James's Hospital, Dublin.

Preface to the second edition

Numerous changes have taken place in acute coronary care since the first edition of this book appeared in 1993, particularly in the area of interventional cardiology. The emphasis in this second edition, however, remains on communicating relevant information to junior hospital staff who are not necessarily skilled in interventional procedures. We have also updated the section dealing with secondary prevention of coronary disease to take stock of recent trial data indicating significant benefit from lipid lowering therapy in terms of reduced total mortality beyond that achieved with dietary advice alone. A new Appendix has been added which allows for rapid calculation of 10-year coronary risk based on an assessment of **total** risk in the context of primary prevention. Evidence based medicine (EBM) footnotes have been added to relevant sections providing data from clinical trials on which some of the therapies and management strategies employed are based. A list of useful references on which the EBM notes are based is also provided in Appendix F.

Preface to the first edition

Myocardial infarction is the greatest single cause of premature death in the western world. Most coronary deaths are due to ventricular fibrillation which is most likely to occur soon after the onset of symptoms. Therefore, all patients suspected of myocardial infarction should be monitored to allow prompt detection and treatment of arrhythmias. Limitation of infarct size by thrombolysis also reduces mortality and morbidity and requires coronary care unit (CCU) facilities. The CCU also provides the opportunity to determine risk factors and initiate management.

This manual is directed at those doctors and nurses involved in patient management in CCUs. It aims to provide a guide to the assessment and management of cardiac patients from their admission to the Accident and Emergency (A&E) department, through their stay in CCU, transfer to a recovery area, and then home. It is hoped that this guide will also be of help to those embarking on CCU management for the first time and to medical students, general practitioners, and to paramedical staff.

ACKNOWLEDGEMENTS

The editors would like to express their sincere appreciation to those who have contributed to this manual. In particular, we would like to thank Dr Binayak Deb who laboured long on the first edition as well as our many colleagues at the Adelaide, Meath and St James's hospitals, Dublin for their advice and guidance in compiling this manual. Dr Gearty, as Lecturer in Postgraduate Cardiology is supported by the Royal City of Dublin Hospital. In addition, we would like to thank Ms Kathleen Kirwan at the Irish Heart Foundation and Ms Teresa Lawlor for their able assistance. We are indebted to the Irish Heart Foundation and to Merck, Sharpe and Dohme Pharmaceuticals for their help in publishing and printing this manual. Finally we are grateful to the European Resuscitation Council for permission to reproduce the algorithm in appendix B and to Academic Press with Professor Kalevi Pyörälä who together granted permission to reproduce the recommendations of the joint TASK FORCE of the ESC/EAS/ESH set out in appendix E.

LIST OF ABBREVIATIONS

A&E	Accident and Emergency
ACE	Angiotensin Converting Enzyme
ACLS	Advanced Cardiac Life Support
AMI	Acute Myocardial Infarction
APTT	Activated Partial Thromboplastin Time
ASMI	Anteroseptal Myocardial Infarction
AV	Atrioventricular
bd	Twice daily
CABG	Coronary Artery Bypass Graft
CCF	Congestive Cardiac Failure
CCU	Coronary Care Unit
CHB	Complete Heart Block
CXR	Chest X-ray
ECG	Electrocardiograph
ECHO	Echocardiography
EBM	Evidence Based Medicine
g	grams
IABP	Intra-aortic Balloon Pump
LBBB	Left Bundle Branch Block
IHD	Ischaemic Heart Disease
iv	Intravenous
JVP	Jugular Venous Pressure
LV	Left Ventricular
mg	milligrams
μg	micrograms
MI	Myocardial Infarction
MR	Mitral Regurgitation/Incompetence
od	Once daily
po	Orally
PTCA	Percutaneous Transluminal Coronary Angioplasty
PVC	Premature Ventricular Contraction
qid	Four times daily

RBBB	Right Bundle Branch Block
RVMI	Right Ventricular Myocardial Infarction
sl	Sublingual
SVT	Supraventricular Tachycardia
tds	Three times daily
TOE	Transoesophageal Echocardiography
VF	Ventricular Fibrillation
V/Q	Ventilation/Perfusion
VSD	Ventricular Septal Defect
VT	Ventricular Tachycardia
U&E	Urea and Electrolytes

1

GENERAL GUIDELINES

PRESENTATION OF ACUTE MYOCARDIAL INFARCTION

Myocardial infarction (MI) is diagnosed by characteristic chest pain with a greater than two-fold rise in cardiac enzymes and typical ECG changes. Particularly in elderly subjects, however, infarction can occur without pain. In the absence of contraindications, all patients with MI should receive thrombolysis as soon as possible and recognition of the characteristic ECG changes listed below is important.

Anterior MI: at least 2mm ST elevation in leads V2–6 (Figures 1(a) and 1(b)).

Anteroseptal MI: at least 2mm ST elevation in leads V2–4 (Figure 2).

Anterolateral MI: at least 2mm ST elevation in leads I, AVL, V2–6 (Figure 3).

Inferior MI: at least 2mm elevation in leads II, III and AVF (Figures 4(a) and 4(b)).

True posterior MI: tall R-wave in V1, and at least 2mm ST depression in leads V2-6 (Figure 5(a) and 5(b)).

Right ventricular MI: at least 2mm ST elevation in right-sided chest leads (Figure 6).

2

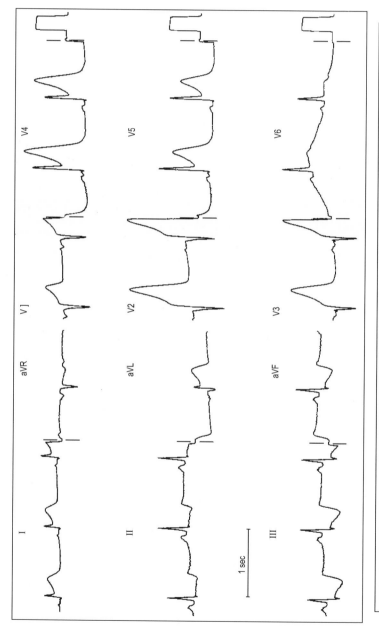

Figure 1(a) Anterior myocardial infarction: ST elevation V2-5. ST depression (reciprocal) L2, 3, AVF.

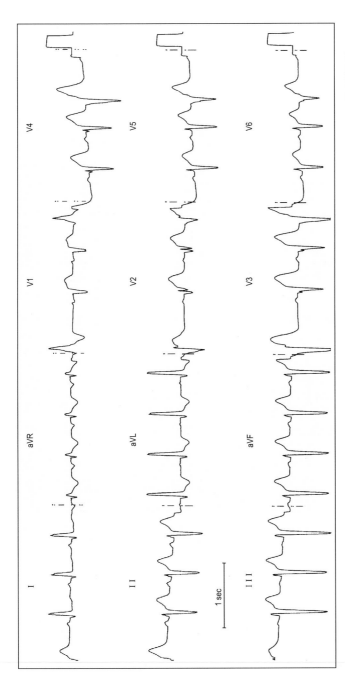

Figure 1(b) Q-wave anterior infarction: sinus tachycardia 100/min; unifocal PVC in V leads. Left axis deviation indicating left anterior hemiblock. Q-wave in V2-4 and ST elevation V2-4.

4

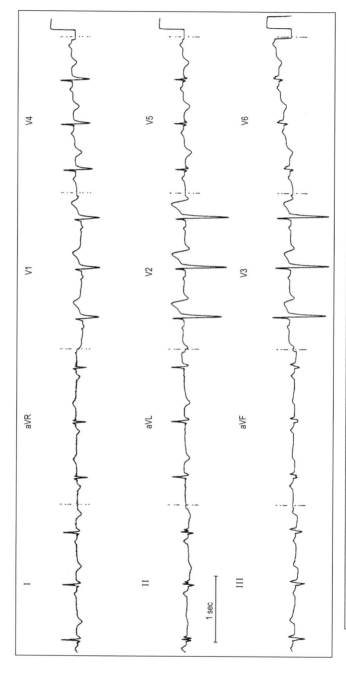

Figure 2 Anteroseptal ischaemia/infarction: biphasic ST segments in V2-4 (probable LAD stenosis).

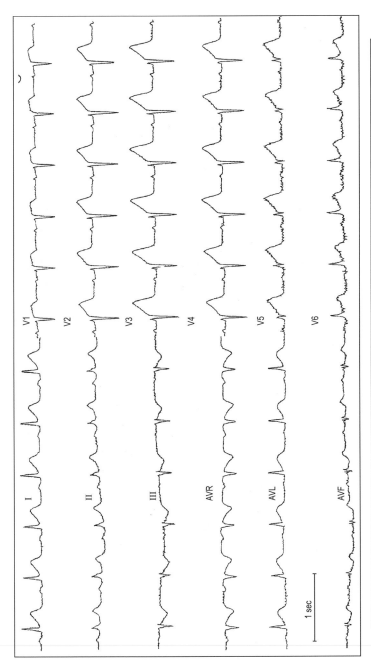

Figure 3 Anterolateral myocardial infarction. ST elevation V2- V6, lead 1 and AVL.

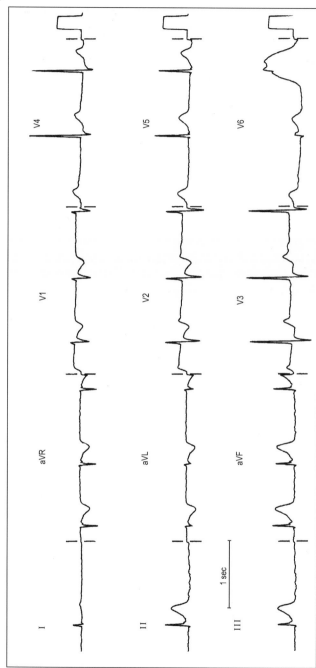

Figure 4(a) Inferior myocardial infarction (right coronary artery occlusion) atrial fibrillation with slow ventricular response 48–70/min; ST elevation L2, 3, AVF, and V6 indicating lateral wall infarction. Note reciprocal ST depression in V1, 2, 3.

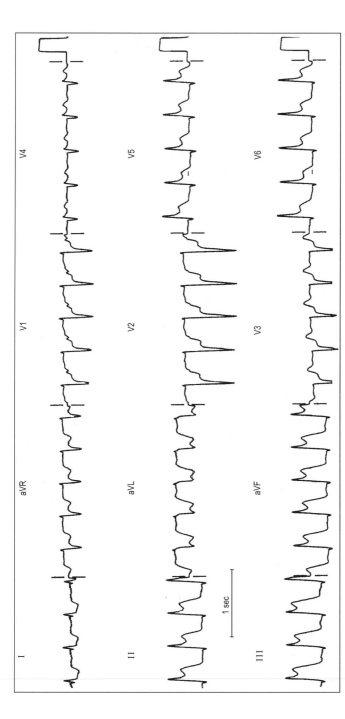

Figure 4(b) Fresh inferior infarction: sinus tachycardia with PR interval (V1) 0.32 sec (first degree AV block). ST elevation LI, III, AVF, V5, V6. ST depression LI, AVL, V1, 2, 3.

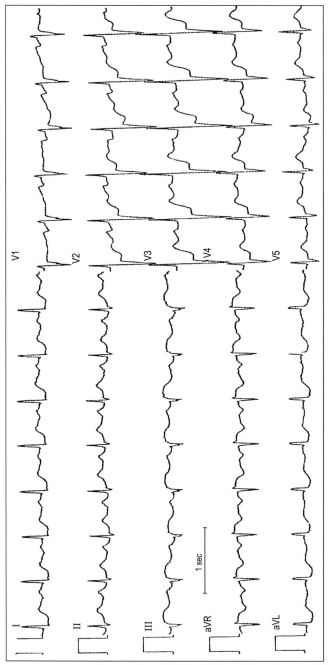

Figure 5(a) True posterior myocardial infarction; R wave in $V_{1,2}$; ST depression anterior leads

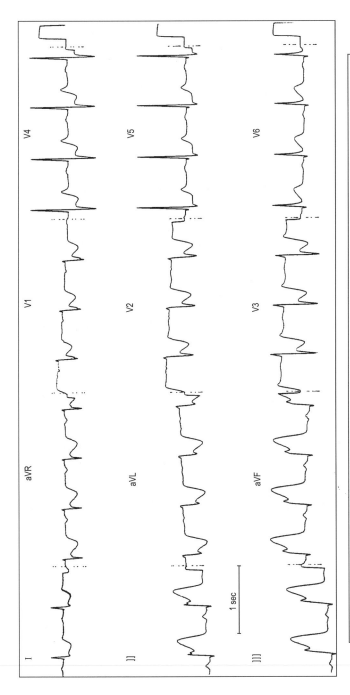

Figure 5(b) Fresh inferior infarction with ST elevation leads, 11, 111 AVF and reciprocal depression leads 1, AVL, V1-V4 suggesting posterior wall extension. Sinus rhythm 90/min.

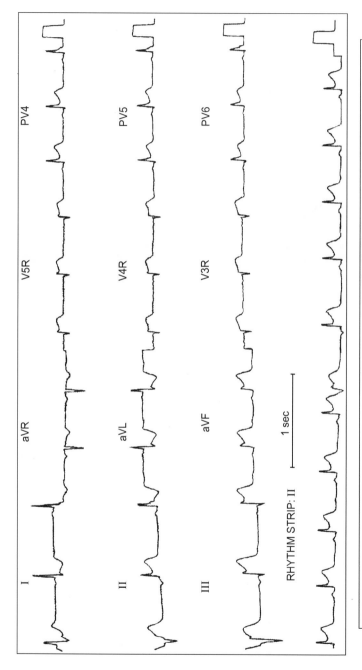

Figure 6 Inferior infarction (ST elevation LII, III, AVF) with right ventricular (ST elevation V3R, V4R, V5R) involvement, sinus bradycardia 60/min. Posterior V leads also demonstrate ST elevation indicating posterior extension of infarction.

INITIAL MANAGEMENT OF ACUTE MI

❯ Accident and Emergency Department

Establish diagnosis	
Take a brief history Examine the patient Perform and interpret 12-lead ECG	Consider thrombolysis inclusion/exclusion criteria

Focus the examination to exclude pulmonary embolism (PE), acute peri-carditis, spontaneous pneumothorax, and aortic dissection. For initial management:

- Give oxygen (100%) at high flow rate, i.e. 10 L/min.
- Give soluble aspirin 150mg po or enteric coated aspirin 300mg to chew.
- Obtain iv access with a cannula and bung; keep open with a saline flush (10ml 8–hourly).
- Give analgesia (cyclimorph 5mg iv and repeat as required).
- Start electrocardiograph (ECG) monitoring.
- Initiate fast-track thrombolysis (as described below).

THROMBOLYSIS

Patients presenting within 12 hours of onset of persisting ischaemic pain and ECG changes consistent with the diagnosis of acute MI should be given thrombolysis without delay. The maximum benefit is in the first 3 hours. The thrombolytic agents commonly used are streptokinase and t-PA.

EBM note: In the 1994 Irish CCU census, 58% of those found to have had myocardial infarction received thrombolysis. The median time from initial symptoms to arrival at hospital was 3 hours for those who had confirmed MI. A further delay of 50 minutes (median) ensued due to hospital administration before admission to CCU. The median time from arrival in CCU to thrombolysis was 25 minutes. These delay times were similar for patients who had a previous history of MI. When given within the first hour after symptom onset, thrombolysis saves 35 lives per thousand patients treated. At 7–12 hours after onset of symptoms, 16 lives per thousand are saved. Operating a fast-track policy where possible is therefore of advantage in reducing the 'door to needle time' and improving prognosis. Equally, educating patients about the nature of coronary symptoms may usefully reduce delay times.

❱ 'Fast-Track' Thrombolysis

The sooner a thrombolytic agent is given in the course of a myocardial infarction the better (Figure 7). Every effort should be made to initiate therapy within 1–2 hours of onset of symptoms. History, examination, ECG and initial assessment should take less than 10 minutes and patients who satisfy the criteria (as listed below), should receive treatment without delay. The 'door to needle time' for patients in

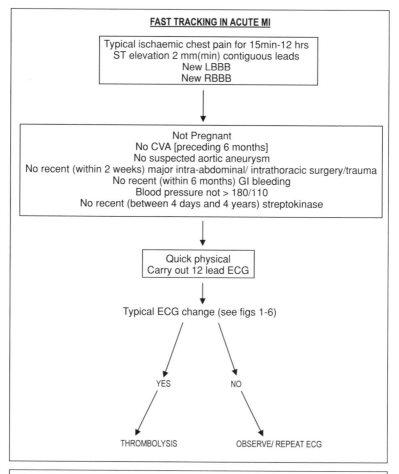

Figure 7 Algorithm for fast-tracking to thrombolysis in acute myocardial infarction.

fast-track should be less than 15 minutes. Thrombolysis should be started in A&E if any delay is expected in transfer to CCU. Investigations such as blood tests and chest X-ray should not delay thrombolysis and neither should temporary pacing for bradycardia or complete heart block.

▶ Indications for thrombolysis

- Acute chest pain.
- Less than 12 hours duration of pain.
- Features of infarction confirmed on the ECG.

▶ Contraindications to thrombolysis

Absolute:
- Active internal bleeding, within previous 6 months.
- Trauma or surgery (within previous 2 weeks).
- Recent head injury or intracranial neoplasm.
- Suspected aortic dissection.
- History of haemorrhagic stroke.
- Pregnancy.

Relative:
- Diabetic haemorrhagic retinopathy.
- Hypertension: blood pressure > 180/110 after iv sedation and/or nitrate.
- Prolonged or traumatic cardiopulmonary resuscitation (CPR).
- Known bleeding diathesis.
- Significant liver disease.
- Non-compressible vascular puncture.

▶ Thrombolysis treatment protocol

Check that soluble aspirin 150mg – 300mg po has been given before thrombolysis. Streptokinase is the thrombolytic of choice. However t-PA is indicated in the following circumstances:

- Patient is a young (<60 years) male with an anterior MI.
- There is a history of allergy to streptokinase.

- Streptokinase given before (4 days – 4 years ago).
- Patient is hypotensive (systolic BP <80mmHg).

Note that streptokinase can be repeated up to 4 days after infarction.

Dose of Streptokinase and t-PA

Streptokinase: reconstitute using 5ml normal saline and dilute to the desired final volume (usually 50–100ml) with normal saline, glucose 5% or Hartmann's solution. Give 1.5 million units in an iv infusion over 60 minutes.

Accelerated regimen of t-PA: reconstitute with solvent provided. This results in a 1mg/ml solution of t-PA. Give a bolus of 15mg (i.e. 15mls of reconstituted solution) iv stat.
Then infuse 50ml over 30 minutes (0.75 ml/kg) followed by 35ml over 60 minutes (0.5ml/kg).

Record ECGs before, during and 2 hours after thrombolysis.
Traditionally heparin has been infused after thrombolysis for at least 24 hours. Evidence to support such treatment is lacking however; see EBM note. Activated Partial Thromboplastin Time (APTT) is maintained at 1.5–2.5 times control. Heparin after t-PA is mandatory because of its short half-life.

EBM note: The evidence favouring the use of heparin is weak and it is questionable whether it should be used. Data from GISSI-2 and ISIS-3 (comparing high dose sc heparin and aspirin with aspirin alone) and GUSTO-1 (comparing iv heparin and aspirin with sc heparin and aspirin) indicate that the addition of heparin to aspirin in patients with acute myocardial infarction provides an early but small added benefit in terms of death, reinfarction or stroke prevention. In high doses heparin increases the risk of significant bleeding. Late (35 day and 6 month) mortality rates are no better in subjects who received heparin. Similarly, in patients with unstable angina no significant benefit is evident. For full discussion see Appendix E for reference: Collins R, Baigent C and Sleight P.

COMPLICATIONS OF THROMBOLYSIS

Bleeding

Intracranial haemorrhage occurs in about 1% of treated patients and is marginally more likely to occur with t-PA than with streptokinase. It is more likely to occur in patients who are elderly (>65 years), female, hypertensive (>180/110) and of low body weight. If this or another form of haemorrhage occurs which is severe, discontinue thrombolytic therapy. Cross match blood and give fresh frozen plasma or cryoprecipitate, or transfuse whole blood if necessary.

Anaphylaxis
- Discontinue thrombolytic therapy.
- Ensure the airway is free.
- Give adrenaline (1ml 1:1000 iv).
- Give iv fluids (hypovolaemia is frequent).
- Give hydrocortisone 200mg iv stat and then 100mg iv 4–6 hourly.

Hypotension
Hypotension is relatively common and usually resolves when the infusion rate is reduced. In severe cases, discontinue thrombolytic therapy and elevate the end of the bed. In some cases, iv fluids and plasma expanders are necessary.

Reperfusion arrhythmias
Premature ventricular contractions (PVCs) and idioventricular dysrhythmias are common and indicate clot lysis in the infarct related artery. Check result of serum K^+ and Mg^{++}. Treat arrhythmias only if symptoms or haemodynamic instability, i.e. dizziness, near syncope or low blood pressure are present.

EBM note: The ISIS-2 trial demonstrated a reduced risk of cardiovascular mortality at 5 weeks, non-fatal myocardial re-infarction, and non-fatal stroke in those randomized to receive aspirin started during the first 24 hours after myocardial infarction. In addition, the trial established the beneficial interaction between streptokinase and aspirin. Thirty-day mortality rates were 10.7% in those given aspirin alone, 10.3% in those given streptokinase alone, 8.0% in those given both and 13.2% in those given neither.

MANAGEMENT OF NON-DIAGNOSTIC ECG CHANGES WITH CHEST PAIN/UNSTABLE ANGINA

Patients who present with a classical history of MI and left bundle branch block (LBBB) on ECG, should not be denied thrombolysis (Figure 8).

In patients with angina lasting more than 30 minutes with minor/non-specific ECG changes, i.e. T-wave inversion/flattening, hyperacute T-waves, non-diagnostic ST segment elevation (Figures 9(a) and 9(b)), the management should include:

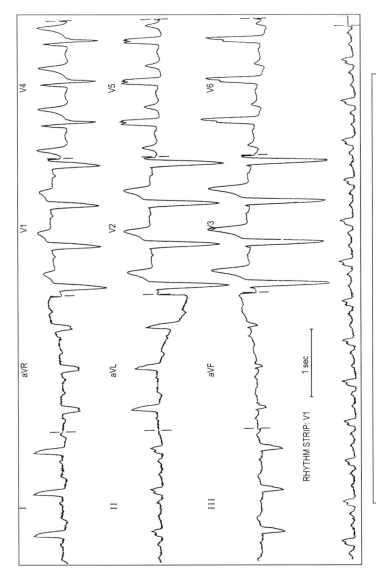

Figure 8 Sinus rhythm with left bundle branch block.

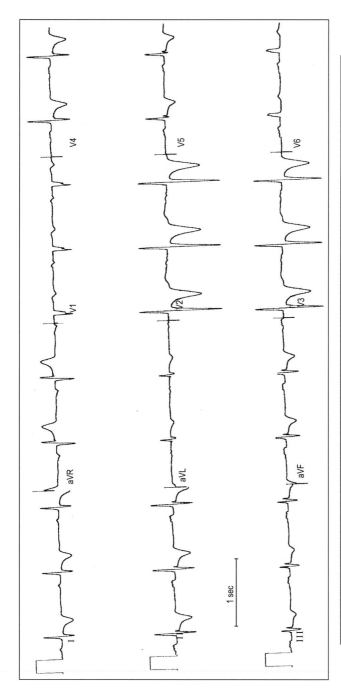

Figure 9(a) Subendocardial myocardial infarction/unstable angina. Sinus rhythm 60/min Deep symmetrical T-wave inversion indicating subendocardial infarction.

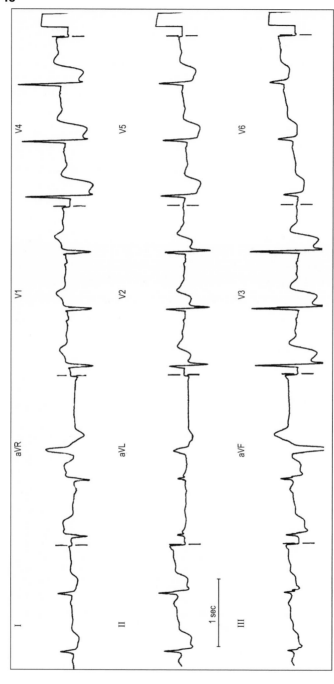

Figure 9(b) Subendocardial infarction. Sinus rhythm, PVC in A leads. Marked 2.5–9 mm ST depression. The patient was found to have advanced 3-vessel disease at angiography.

- Aspirin (if no contraindication) 150mg – 300mg po.
- Oxygen 100% at 10 L/min via mask or nasal prongs.
- Analgesia (cyclimorph 5mg iv and repeated as necessary).
- Intravenous nitrates (assuming the exclusion of right ventricular infarction).
- Intravenous heparin (assuming no contraindication).
- Repeat ECG every 15–30 minutes until pain and ECG changes settle or diagnostic changes occur.
- When diagnostic changes occur, consider thrombolysis promptly (in the absence of contraindications).

In cases of persistent pain without ECG evidence of evolving MI, check for pulmonary embolism, aortic dissection, respiratory tract infection, peptic ulcer, gastro-oesophageal reflux, costochondritis, cholecystitis and pneumothorax.

The emphasis is on ensuring adequate analgesia and haemodynamic stability followed by a systematic review of the differential diagnoses. Patients with persistent cardiac pain and ECG changes of MI which fail to settle after thrombolysis should be considered for early coronary angiography with a view to angioplasty.

2

MANAGEMENT OF MYOCARDIAL INFARCTION IN THE CCU

ADMISSION POLICY

Patients with suspected acute MI who present within the first 24 hours, or with unstable angina, potentially serious arrhythmias, or severe heart failure should be admitted to the CCU.

The atmosphere in CCU should be one of reassuring tranquility. Patients who are resting or sleeping should not be woken for routine observations if they are clearly haemodynamically stable. The likely diagnosis and all procedures and treatments should be clearly explained. Such explanations may need to be repeated because pain and anxiety impair comprehension. Ideally, a full explanation should be given to relatives or close companions. It should also be stressed that most patients recover and lead normal lives and that the process of rehabilitation and patient education starts immediately.

Therapeutic measures initiated in A&E are continued in CCU. Oxygen at high concentration (100% at 10 L/min) is given at least in the initial hours for all patients with acute ischaemic pain except in cases of chronic obstructive airways disease where lower concentrations (24–28%) are used. Ensure adequate analgesia. For severe pain, give morphine sulphate 5mg iv or diamorphine 2.5–5.0mg iv and repeat as required. Slow iv injection gives more rapid and predictable effect. Metoclopramide 10mg iv may be given in conjuction as an antiemetic. Cyclimorph 5mg iv can also be given. However, each ampoule contains 50mg of cyclizine and the maximum recommended dose of cyclizine in 24 hours is 150mg.

For milder pain give glyceryl trinitrate 0.5mg tab or spray sl as required. For persistent ischaemic pain which is associated with ST segment depression, commence an isosorbide dinitrate infusion and titrate the dose against the analgesic response and blood pressure (Appendix A shows regimen).

Long-acting nitrates or a buccal formulation may be used when the patient is further stabilized. Cardioselective beta-blockers may be used particularly for those with sinus tachycardia or hypertension without heart failure. The treatment strategy is:

- Ensure all patients have 2 venous cannulae and bungs. Keep cannulae patent with saline flush/heparinized saline (10ml 8-hourly).
- Continue ECG monitoring until stable.
- Record ECG daily and during episodes of pain.
- Obtain a portable chest X-ray (CXR) on admission and a full PA film as soon as the patient is fit to go to the X-ray department.
- Send blood for full blood count, urea and electrolytes (U&E), Mg^{++}, cardiac enzymes (including MB fraction) and coagulation screen on admission if not already sent from A&E.
- Send U&E and cardiac enzymes daily for the first three days.
- Send blood for fasting lipid profile and blood sugar within the first 24 hours.

3

RIGHT VENTRICULAR INFARCTION

Right ventricular MI (RVMI) (Figure 6), is more common than previously thought. It may occur in isolation or in association with up to half of all inferior MIs. A high index of suspicion is required and right-sided ECG V leads should be recorded in all cases of suspected inferior infarction to look for ST elevation over the right ventricle. Leads V3 and 4 are placed at the same intercostal space as usual but to the right side of the sternum. Look for ST segment elevation. Such changes may be transient and an early ECG is required. The main reason for making this specific diagnosis is because therapy differs from that for pure left ventricular MI. The clinical triad of hypotension, raised venous pressure and clear lung fields should suggest the diagnosis bearing in mind that hypovolaemia may mask the signs. Other signs which may co-exist but which are not essential for the diagnosis are Kussmaul's sign, a right ventricular gallop, tricuspid regurgitation and AV dissociation.

The therapeutic strategy should be to increase right ventricular preload to maintain cardiac output, reduce right ventricular afterload, provide inotropic support for the right ventricle, and reperfuse the infarct-related artery. Apart from the measures below, the treatment strategies as outlined in Chapters 1 and 2 apply.

- Avoid diuretics and negative inotropic agents.
- Several litres of fluid may be required. In some, the right ventricular pressure may increase further with no improvement in cardiac output. In such cases, inotropic support with dobutamine is indicated. If invasive monitoring is available, aim for a pulmonary capillary wedge pressure of 15mmHg.
- Consider AV sequential pacing.
- DC cardiovert promptly if atrial fibrillation occurs.
- Where left ventricular dysfunction occurs in association with right ventricular MI, consider the use of sodium nitroprusside and/or an intra-aortic counterpulsation device.

- Give aspirin and thrombolysis early as with all MIs.
- Consider angioplasty to reopen the infarct-related artery if symptoms and ECG changes do not settle following thrombolysis.

4

Post-myocardial infarction angina

Thrombolytic therapy lyses the acute thrombus formed over the ruptured atheromatous plaque in the coronary artery. The plaque may, by itself, be large enough to cause significant stenosis of the vascular lumen and hence angina even after thrombolysis has achieved reperfusion. Angina occurring at rest, or on minimal exertion, in the post-infarction period is an indication for further aggressive investigation and treatment. Typically the cardiac enzyme assays are normal and ECGs show non-specific T-wave flattening or inversion along with ST segment depression, or, in some cases, ST segment elevation.

Management includes intravenous heparin, nitrates and sometimes beta antagonists, followed by oral nitrates with or without beta antagonists, when the acute episode has settled. Calcium channel antagonists, particularly those with long half-lives, are also effective agents. Unstable angina in the peri-and post-infarction period is a strong indication for early coronary angiography to define coronary artery anatomy and plan further therapy and interventions based on this knowledge.

5

LIPIDS − POST-MYOCARDIAL INFARCTION MANAGEMENT

All patients with suspected MI should have a fasting lipid profile taken within 24 hours of admission (later samples may be falsely low). General dietary advice regarding salt, fat, protein, and carbohydrate intake should be provided to all patients. Specific strict dietary measures should be instituted for patients with significantly high total cholesterol levels (>5.2 mmol/L) and institution of drug treatment should be considered for post-MI patients who have had previously raised total cholesterol levels despite the implementation of dietary advice. A low HDL cholesterol level (<1.0 mmol/L) and the presence of other risk factors such as smoking or hypertension greatly increase the risk associated with an elevated total cholesterol (appendix E) and lower the threshold for drug treatment of hypercholesterolaemia.

EBM note: Recent trials have shown a 20–30% relative risk reduction in all cause and cardiovascular mortality in both primary (WOSCOPS) and secondary prevention (4S and CARE) settings using statins. See Chapter 10 and Appendix F for references.

6

FOLLOW UP TREATMENT POST-MYOCARDIAL INFARCTION

Aspirin

A dose of 75mg soluble aspirin daily or 300mg enteric coated aspirin on alternate days should be routinely prescribed unless the patient has active reflux oesophagitis, active peptic ulcer disease or allergy to aspirin.

Beta-antagonists

Proven to reduce post-infarct morbidity and mortality by preventing arrhythmias, cardiac rupture, controlling blood pressure and reducing myocardial workload and oxygen demand. Should be considered for all patients post-MI in the absence of contraindications.

Angiotensin Converting Enzyme (ACE) Inhibitors

When prescribed 24–48 hours post-infarct, may help to reduce remodelling of ventricular myocardium and perhaps arrhythmias, thereby reducing overall morbidity and mortality. Also effective in patients with clinical or echocardiographic (ECHO) evidence of congestive cardiac failure (CCF) post-infarction. Start at lowest possible dose and increase to maximum tolerated dose, while monitoring symptoms, blood pressure and renal function. First dose hypotension may occur, but is not necessarily an indication for stopping ACE inhibitor therapy.

Nitrates

Oral, sublingual or patches are prescribed to relieve angina. In patients with mild CCF, nitrates can reduce preload and hence improve exercise tolerance and symptoms. It is important to ensure a 6–8 hour nitrate-free period in each 24 hours to avoid nitrate tolerance. Hence, for patients with early morning angina, nitrates are best administered at bedtime to offer protection in the early morning hours. This would provide a nitrate-free period in the afternoon on the following day. Sublingual nitrate may be used prior to anticipated exertion to prevent angina. Nitrates in any form can cause significant postural hypotension and headaches. Patients should be warned about these. Paracetamol can be used for headaches.

Calcium Channel Antagonists

Diltiazem is commonly used for post-infarct angina. Other long-acting agents are also good for symptom control. They are especially useful in patients with angina, hypertension and beta-antagonist intolerance. There is no evidence to date that calcium channel antagonists improve prognosis.

Anticoagulants

Warfarin may reduce the likelihood of thrombo-embolic complications in patients with large infarcts, mural thrombi, dilated cardiomyopathy, post-infarction atrial fibrillation, deep vein thrombosis or pulmonary embolism.

7

COMPLICATIONS OF MYOCARDIAL INFARCTION

CARDIAC DYSRHYTHMIAS

Sinus Tachycardia (Figure 10)

Check for and treat the underlying cause such as associated heart failure, pulmonary embolism, pain, anxiety or the effect of nitrates. Coincidental infection should be excluded. Small doses of beta-antagonists may be tried to reduce sympathetic tone especially if blood pressure is high.

Sinus Bradycardia (Figures 11(a) and (b))

This may occur transiently due to pain or anxiety. It is common with inferior wall infarctions, calcium channel blockers and beta-antagonists including eye-drop formulations.

Treatment is advised if the bradycardia is associated with symptoms or hypotension. Give atropine 1mg iv and repeat if needed. If bradycardia continues to be a problem, insert a temporary pacemaker. Alternatively, where a transvenous pacemaker cannot be readily inserted, or a transcutaneous pacemaker is unavailable, try isoprenaline by infusion $2–20\mu g/$ min.

Atrial Ectopics (Figure 12)

These do not require treatment.

Paroxysmal Supraventricular Tachycardia (Figures 13(a), (b) and (c))

This may cause hypotension. First line measures include carotid sinus pressure although this is not ideal in elderly patients and may cause further lowering of blood pressure. In the context of patients with myocardial infarction, it is not recommended that the Valsalva manoeuvre be used.

- Adenosine 6mg iv as first line medication may be given as a **rapid** bolus. If unsuccessful, give further boluses of 6mg, 12mg and 18mg. (Warn the patient that he/she will experience chest pain and ensure

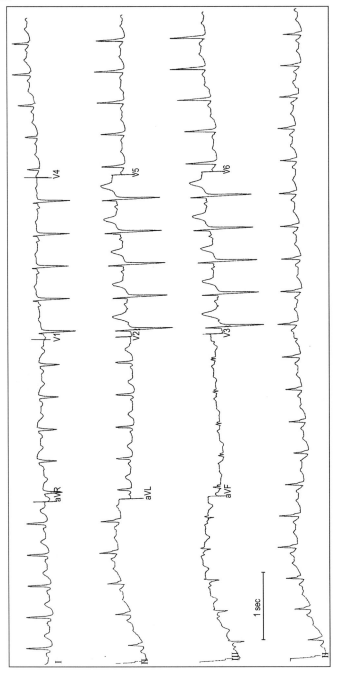

Figure 10 Sinus tachycardia, 120/min.

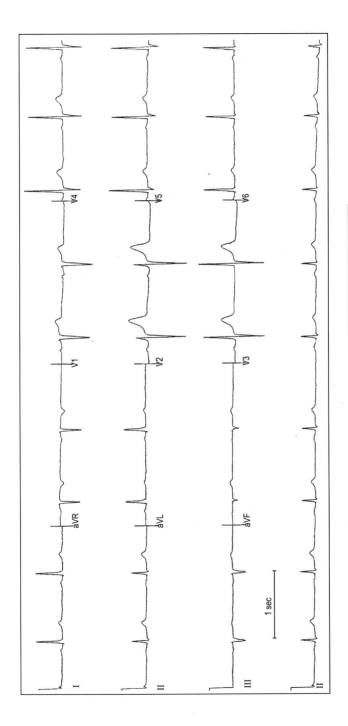

Figure 11(a) Sinus bradycardia, 55/min.

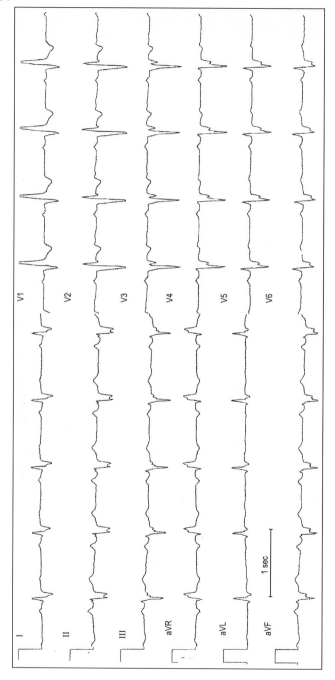

I
II
III
aVR
aVL
aVF

V1
V2
V3
V4
V5
V6

1 sec

Figure 11(b) Sinus bradycardia, right bundle branch block, old anteroseptal MI.

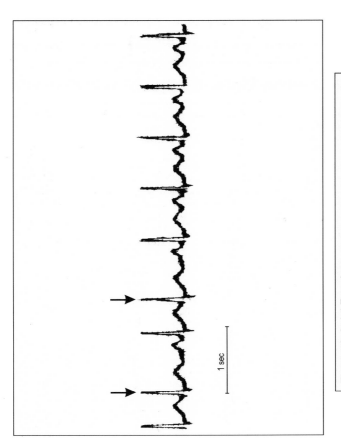

Figure 12 Atrial Ectopics.

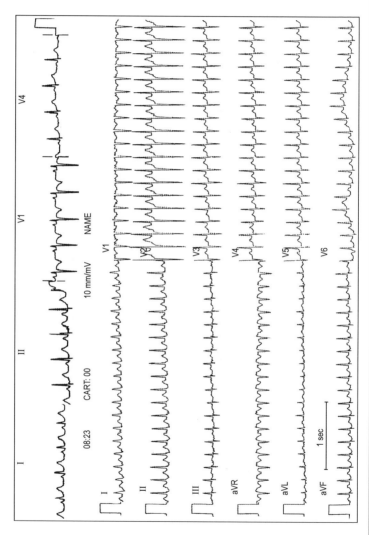

Figure 13(a) Top: Sinus rhythm. Bottom: Regular tachycardia 200/min. Normal QRS. Small retrograde P in lead II and VI.

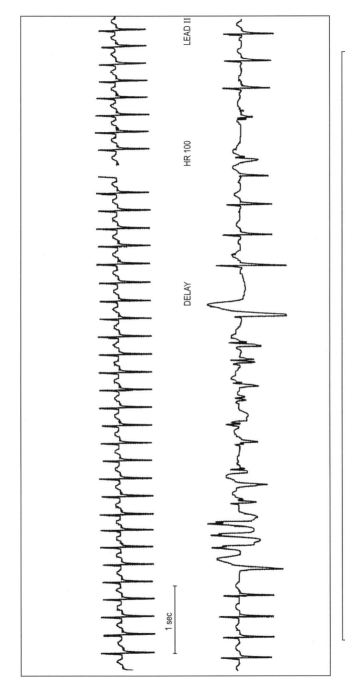

Figure 13(b) Paroxysmal nodal SVT. Regular tachycardia 220/min. Normal QRS. Adenosine 6mg iv given followed by ventricular ectopics and sinus rhythm.

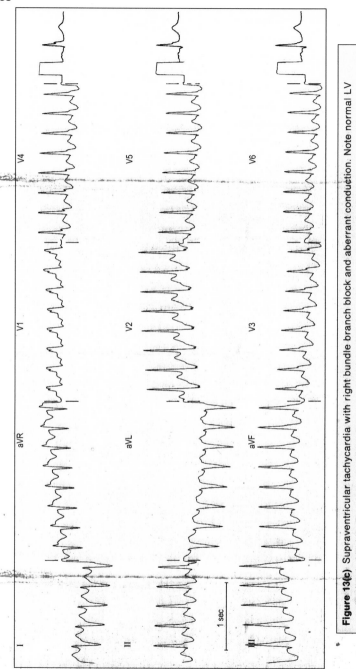

Figure 13(c) Supraventricular tachycardia with right bundle branch block and aberrant conduction. Note normal LV conduction in V5, V6. Far right, leads V4–6: return to sinus rhythm.

that the patient is not taking dipyridamole or theophylline and does not suffer from asthma.)

- Verapamil 5–10mg iv rapidly if adenosine is unsuccessful. Repeat this dose after 5 minutes if necessary (maximum recommended dose is 20mg). Verapamil may cause hypotension especially in subjects with already impaired LV function.

- Amiodarone as a bolus may be given in a dose of 5mg/kg in 100ml 5% dextrose over 20 minutes. This should be followed by a maintenance infusion of 900–1200mg in 5% dextrose over 24 hours via a central line.

- Beta-antagonists such as atenolol 5mg iv may be tried but do not give with verapamil because of the risk of asystole. It should also be given with caution in patients taking digoxin. Esmolol, a short acting beta-1 antagonist given as an infusion, may be useful in controlling SVT and can be titrated safely against its effect because of its short half-life.

- DC shock should be tried in cases which prove resistant to medical treatment, especially where ventricular function is impaired and negatively inotropic agents are to be avoided.

Atrial Flutter and Fibrillation (Figures 14(a) (b) and (c))

Atrial fibrillation is more likely to occur with large infarcts, anterior infarcts, in subjects with congestive heart failure, and may also occur in subjects with right ventricular infarction (occlusion of artery to sinoatrial node). The treatment strategy is as below:

- Digitalize orally if haemodynamically stable; 0.5mg stat, then 0.25mg 6-hourly for 12 hours followed by a maintenance dose of 0.0625mg–0.25mg daily po.

- If haemodynamically unstable, or if rapid control is desirable an iv loading dose of 0.5mg–1.0mg digoxin in 50ml of normal saline or 5% dextrose over 20 minutes, followed by a maintenance of 0.0625mg–0.25mg daily po. Individualize the dose and reduce as appropriate in subjects with renal failure and in the elderly.

- If inadequate control is achieved, give verapamil, 5–10mg slowly iv or 40–160mg tds po or beta-antagonists, e.g. atenolol 5mg iv or 50–100mg po monitoring blood pressure and LV function.

N.B.: *IV verapamil should not be given together with an IV beta-antagonist because of the risk of asystole and hypotension.*

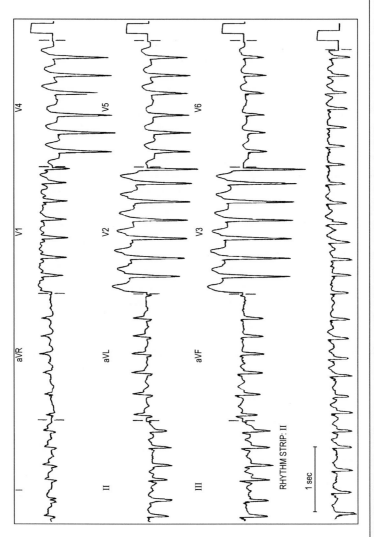

Figure 14(a) Atrial fibrillation. Irregular tachycardia 140–180/min. Ischaemic features: QST patterns in lead I, AVL, V4-6 consistent with old anterolateral infarction with aneurysm formation.

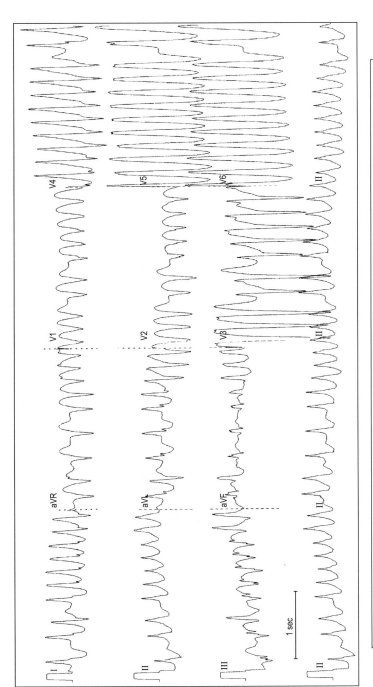

Figure 14(b) Atrial fibrillation. Irregular tachycardia 160- 280/min. Broad variable QRS and pre-excitation syndrome likely.

42

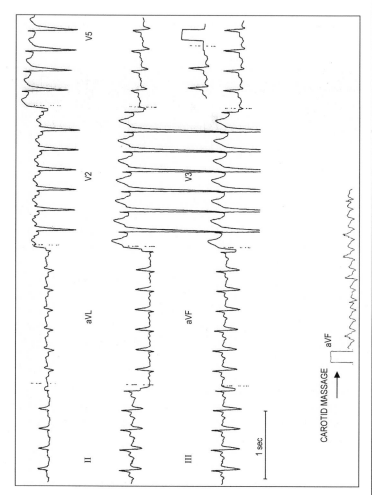

Figure 14(c) Atrial flutter. Regular tachycardia 150–160/min. Normal QRS. Flutter patterns leads II, III, AVF, and VI. Bottom: Carotid massage increases AV block and slows ventricular conduction.

- Amiodarone may be given by central line in cases resistant to other medical therapies. In a proportion of cases cardioversion to sinus rhythm is achieved. The regimen used is as outlined above for treatment of SVT.
- Synchronized DC shock, 50–100 J for atrial flutter and 200–360 J for atrial fibrillation in resistant cases or those showing rapid haemodynamic deterioration.
- Those with persistent atrial fibrillation should be anticoagulated. Heparinize if atrial fibrillation occurs in the context of acute MI assuming no contraindication.

Ventricular Ectopics (Figures 15(a) and (b))

Correct the underlying cause if possible, e.g. hypokalaemia, hypomagnesaemia, hypo-or hypercalcaemia, drugs such as digoxin, sympathomimetics, and tricyclic antidepressants. Ventricular ectopics should be treated if they are **frequent, multifocal or show R on T salvoes**, as they may lead to ventricular fibrillation (VF). However, VF (Figure 16), frequently occurs unheralded. If ventricular ectopics are associated with sinus bradycardia, atropine may be indicated as they often disappear when the heart rate is accelerated. Other types of ventricular ectopics do not normally require treatment.

Treatment options include lignocaine 50–100mg as an iv bolus over 2 minutes followed by a maintenance infusion of 1–4 mg/min. The infusion may be reduced after 24 hours or sooner if the patient is elderly or has impaired liver function. If this fails, disopyramide as a 2mg/kg bolus given over 5 minutes followed by an infusion of 0.4mg/kg/hr may be tried.

Ventricular fibrillation (Figure 16)

The emphasis in treating confirmed VF is on early defibrillation. Use unsynchronized DC shock 200J and repeat shocks at energies of 200J and 360J, as shown in Appendix B.

Ventricular tachycardia

Ventricular tachycardia (VT) (Figures 17a and 17b), is defined as runs of three or more consecutive ventricular ectopic beats. The treatment strategy is given below, however, short runs with no hemodynamic compromise may not need treatment.

Treatment is by synchronized DC shock if the patient is haemodynamically compromised; start at 200J, repeat at 200J and again at 360J if

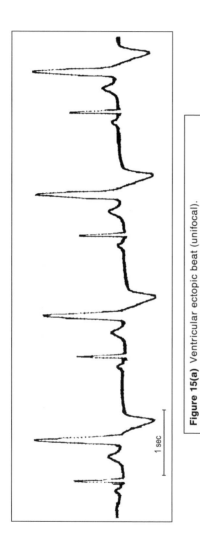

Figure 15(a) Ventricular ectopic beat (unifocal).

1 sec

Figure 15(b) Ventricular ectopic beat (multifocal).

1 sec

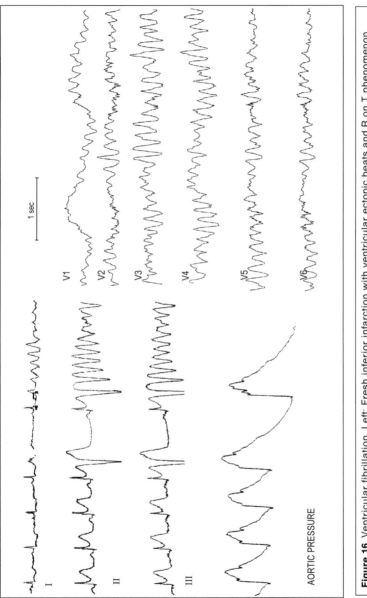

Figure 16 Ventricular fibrillation. Left: Fresh inferior infarction with ventricular ectopic beats and R on T phenomenon followed by ventricular fibrillation. Right: Ventricular fibrillation. Note drop in aortic pressure with onset of VF.

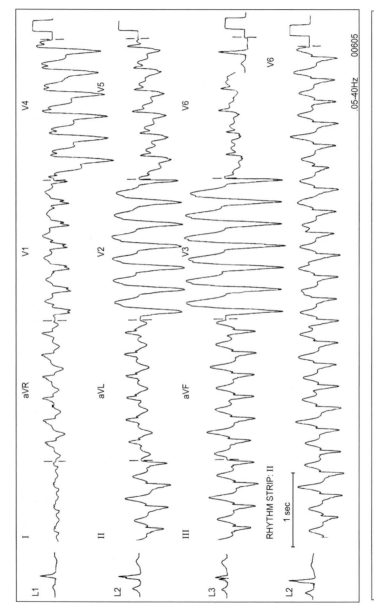

Figure 17(a) Ventricular tachycardia. Regular, broad complex tachycardia with extreme left axis deviation. Tracings at extreme right and left indicate baseline QRST morphology for different leads.

.05-40Hz   00605

47

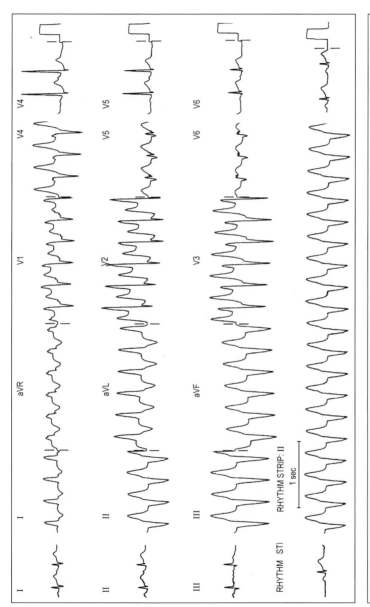

Figure 17(b) Ventricular tachycardia. Regular, broad complex tachycardia, 150/min with extreme left axis deviation. Tracings at extreme right and left indicate baseline QRST morphology for different leads.

necessary. Light sedation (e.g. midazolam 10mg) should be given prior to the procedure if the patient is conscious. Successful cardioversion is then followed by suppressive therapy, as below. If the patient is not haemodynamically compromised, suppressive therapy on its own can be tried:

- Lignocaine may be given as in the regimen for ventricular ectopics.
- Disopyramide, may be given as in the regimen for ventricular ectopics.
- Amiodarone 5mg/kg iv bolus over 30 minutes followed by an infusion of 900–1200mg iv over 24 hours via a central line.
- Overdrive/underdrive pacing can be tried if the above measures fail.

Broad complex tachycardia

The differential diagnosis includes ventricular tachycardia (VT) and supraventricular tachycardia (SVT) with aberrant conduction. Points in favour of a diagnosis of VT are:

- AV dissociation.
- Capture or fusion beats.
- QRS duration > 140 (m/sec.)
- Extreme left axis deviation.
- Rsr pattern in V1 and/or QS or rS pattern in V6.
- Ventricular concordance, i.e. QRS complex is either positive or negative in all chest leads.

First line treatment is DC shock as for the treatment of VT if the patient is haemodynamically unstable. Similarly, if the diagnosis is in doubt, treat as for VT. If the diagnosis is one of SVT with aberrant conduction, give adenosine 6mg as an iv bolus. Warn the patient that chest pain will be experienced with adenosine. This has no effect on VT. The half-life of adenosine is short and the dose can be repeated up to doses of 18mg. Verapamil should not be given in VT as worsening of hypotension will ensue.

▶ AV Conduction Defects

First degree AV block (Figure 18a)

No treatment is required

Second degree AV block

Mobitz type I or the Wenckebach phenomenon (Figure 18(b)) is characterized by progressive prolongation of the PR interval until a P-wave is no longer conducted: usually no treatment is required.

Mobitz Type II (Figure 18(c)) is characterized by a fixed PR interval with a non-conducted P-wave occurring at intervals. When this occurs in the context of an inferior wall MI, a temporary pacemaker may be needed if there is haemodynamic compromise. In anterior wall infarction, temporary pacing is almost mandatory because of the risk of progression to third degree AV block or asystole.

Third degree AV block (Figure 18d$_1$ d$_2$ and d$_3$)

Temporary pacing is indicated in anterior wall MI irrespective of the presence of symptoms because of the risk of asystole. In inferior wall infarcts, if the patient is stable, pacing may be deferred.

Bradycardias

These may be due to concomitant illness, e.g. hypothyroidism or medications, e.g. beta-antagonists, digoxin or calcium antagonsits. First, second and third (complete) degree heart block commonly occur in the peri-infarction period especially with inferior infarction. In this situation, bradycardias tend to be transient and resolve spontaneously. However, if the bradycardia is associated with hypotension and/or near syncope, atropine 0.6–1.2mg iv may help until a temporary pacemaker is inserted. Heart block associated with anterior infarction signifies greater myocardial damage and poorer prognosis. Such patients need early temporary pacemaker insertion.

ACUTE PULMONARY OEDEMA AND CARDIOGENIC SHOCK

The appearance of dyspnoea, tachypnoea, tachycardia with or without hypotension, a third heart sound and pulmonary crackles suggest myocardial dysfunction leading to accumulation of fluid in the pulmonary circulation (Figure 19). The signs and symptoms may be transient (myocardial stunning) in the early post-infarct period. Management of **acute pulmonary oedema** includes:

- Sit the patient up.
- Humidified oxygen in high concentration (100%). If pulmonary disease is present, use a lower concentration of oxygen.

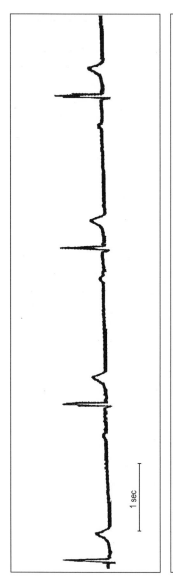

Figure 18(a) First degree heart block. PR interval 0.3 sec.

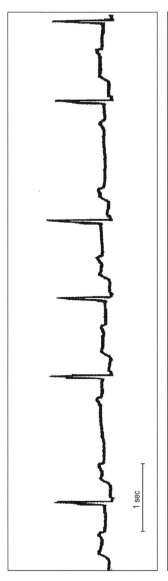

Figure 18(b) Second degree heart block (Wenckebach). Every fourth P-wave is not conducted to the ventricle. Progressive prolongation of the PR interval occurs before the non-conducted P-wave appears.

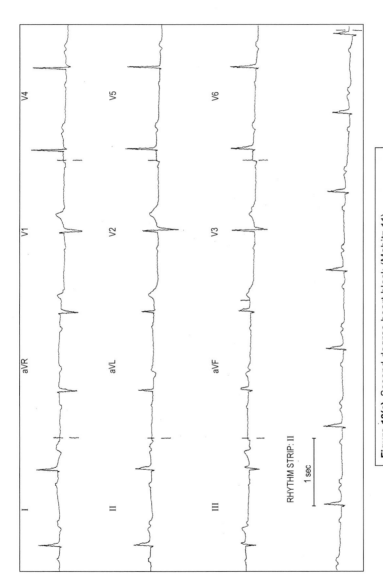

Figure 18(c) Second degree heart block (Mobitz 11).

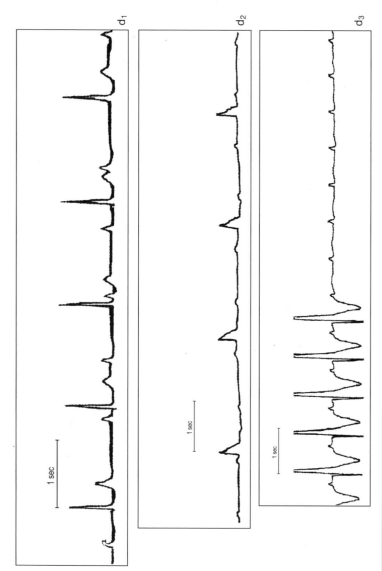

Figure 18(d₁) Third degree heart block at AV nodal level. No constant PR interval noted. Ventricular rhythm is regular with a rate of 44/min. QRS comlexes are narrow indicating high AV block. (**d₂**) Third degree heart block at ventricular level. Slow ventricular rate at 38/min. Wide QRS complexes indicating low level block. (**d₃**) Third degree heart block of abrupt onset. Patient had an acute anterior M1, developed right bundle branch block and complete heart block ensued. No ventricular escape rhythm present indicating ventricular asystole.

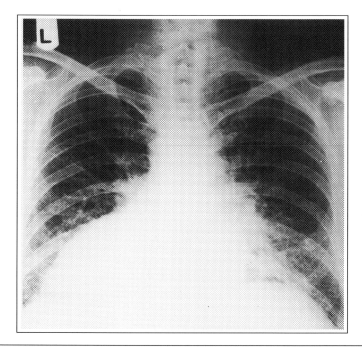

Figure 19 Acute pulmonary oedema.

- Frusemide 40–80mg iv.
- Morphine 3mg iv slowly (with repeated dosing if necessary) or diamorphine 2.5–10mg iv. Respiratory depression may occur with high doses which may be reversed by naloxone 0.4mg iv (up to a maximum of 3 doses).

A venodilator which reduces pre-load (venous return) such as an iv nitrate can be given. Inotropic support such as dobutamine, and/or positive pressure ventilation may be required in severe cases.

Bedside echocardiography (if available) helps to assess ventricular size and overall function. CXR helps to confirm the clinical diagnosis. Fluid restriction to prevent overload may be instituted.

In resistant/severe cardiac failure not responding to the above medications with hypotension (systolic <90mmHg or a drop in 30mmHg compared to basal levels) **or** oliguria/anuria and poor tissue perfusion **or** elevated left heart filling pressures in the absence of hypovolaemia and right ventricular myocardial infarction, the diagnosis is one of **cardiogenic shock** and the treatment includes inotropic support:

- Dobutamine starting at $2.5\mu g/kg/min$ and titrated observing the BP and pulse response.
- Alternatively dopamine can be used but a central venous line is needed. Dosage starts at $2.5\mu g/kg/min$ and is titrated upwards according to the haemodynamic response.

Other inotropes available are dopexamine (Dopacard) and adrenaline/noradrenaline, the doses for which are listed in Appendix A. Dopexamine may be a better choice if myocardial oxygen demand is at a premium.

Patients in **cardiogenic shock** should have a Swan Ganz catheter inserted to allow assessment of right and left heart pressures, cardiac output, and easier titration of the doses of medications used. Patients also need urinary catheterization to assess intake and output balance. Echocardiography helps to exclude mechanical complications of infarction (ventricular septal defect, rupture of the free wall of the left ventricle, mitral regurgitation, cardiac tamponade) as a cause of shock.

Consider non-cardiac causes, e.g. pulmonary embolism, hypovolaemia, abdominal aortic aneurysm rupture.

Management includes

- High-flow oxygen by mask, or intubate and ventilate.
- Relieve pain.
- Cardiovert to restore sinus rhythm if a malignant dysrhythmia is present.
- Vasodilate where left heart pressures are high, e.g. acute valvular regurgitation.
- Consider (where available) PTCA to open the infarct-related artery.

An intra-aortic balloon pump can sustain patients with cardiogenic shock. Usually, it is only indicated when there is surgically correctable cause of the shock.

EBM note: Few studies and no randomized controlled trials have been carried out testing the value of PTCA or intra-aortic balloon pumping against supportive management and those which have were on highly selected subjects.

RUPTURE OF VENTRICULAR FREE WALL

Rupture of the ventricle is more likely to occur in first infarcts, large transmural infarcts, or anterior infarcts. It is more common in women, the elderly, and where collateral blood supply to the infarcted area is likely to be poor. Such subjects may have no previous history of angina. The features and initial management are those of cardiogenic shock with generally poor prognosis. Surgical treatment can salvage occasional cases.

ACUTE MITRAL INCOMPETENCE

Acute mitral incompetence (Figure 20), resulting from papillary muscle dysfunction or rupture can lead to cardiogenic shock. Clinically, sudden onset of pulmonary oedema with a new harsh mitral incompetence murmur in the peri-infarction period should suggest the diagnosis, which can be confirmed by echocardiography. An aggressive management approach with ventilation, balloon pumping and surgical treatment should be adopted.

ACUTE VENTRICULAR SEPTAL DEFECT

Acute ventricular septal defect (Figure 21), resulting from MI presents with shock and examination may reveal a pansystolic murmur and praecordial thrill and signs of CCF. Management includes early echocardiography for diagnosis, insertion of a Swan Ganz catheter and inotropic support for shock. Some patients may require intra-aortic balloon pumping as a temporary measure prior to emergency corrective surgery or rarely, may survive the event with conservative management.

LEFT VENTRICULAR ANEURYSM

Left ventricular aneurysm (Figure 22), is more likely after large transmural infarction. Echocardiography and LV angiogram help to make the diagnosis. Management includes, treatment of heart failure, arrhythmias and anticoagulation for prevention of thromboembolic events. Indications for surgical treatment include continual angina pectris, resistant rhythm disturbances and occasionally heart failure.

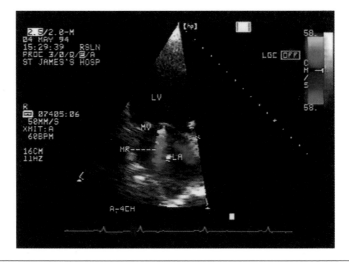

Figure 20 Colour flow mapping in the apical four-chamber view showing the blue jet of retrograde flow (MR) in mitral regurgitation.

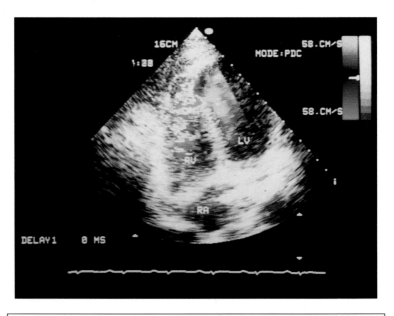

Figure 21 Ventricular septal defect indicated by colour flow doppler.

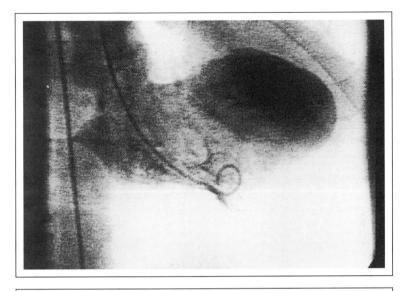

Figure 22 Chest X-ray demonstrating left ventricular aneurysm at angiography.

PERICARDITIS

Pericarditis occurs early but not usually within the first 24 hours, usually without haemodynamic compromise, and it resolves spontaneously. It may require analgesia such as high-dose aspirin or indomethacin. Pericarditis, pleurisy, and a pyrexia with raised white cell count and ESR appearing 2–6 weeks post-MI constitute Dressler's Syndrome. Treatment includes analgesia with indomethacin 25–50mg three times daily. Some patients may require steroids.

DEEP VEIN THROMBOSIS AND PULMONARY EMBOLISM

Deep vein thrombosis and pulmonary embolism are rare events post-infarction. Prevention is achieved with early mobilization, physiotherapy and use of subcutaneous heparin in the peri-infarction period. Pleuritic chest pain, unexplained tachycardia, hypoxia and disproportionate dyspnoea are clinical signs of pulmonary embolism. Management is with heparin 5000–10 000 units iv bolus followed by 1000 units/hr maintaining the APTT 1.5–2.5 times control. Venography and/or V/Q scanning may be necessary to confirm diagnosis. Concomitant warfarin therapy is initiated and continued for 3–6 months.

8

INTERVENTIONS

PERCUTANEOUS TRANSLUMINAL CORONARY ANGIOPLASTY (PTCA)

Availability limited to specialized centres, PTCA may be indicated in:

1. Stable angina pectoris especially where a culprit stenosis can be identified (elective PTCA).
2. Unstable angina('Bail Out' PTCA).
3. Evolving MI where thrombolysis is contraindicated (Primary PTCA).
4. After thrombolysis where symptoms/other evidence of ischaemia persist.

See also cardiogenic shock in Chapter 7

COMPLICATIONS

1. Restenosis in ~ 30% of patients: repeat PTCA of such patients achieves ~ 80% overall success.
2. Abrupt closure of vessel at site of plaque (<5%).
3. MI (<3%).
4. Emergency coronary artery bypass graft (CABG) (<2%).

MANAGEMENT

Careful patient selection and balloon sizing, optimal pre-, peri-and post-procedural anticoagulation and vasodilation (iv/ic nitrates) will minimize early complications. Later complications, namely restenosis which manifest as recurrent angina may be dealt with by a second PTCA. Coronary stenting is playing an increasing role in the management of acute MI.

EBM note: Available evidence suggests that patients with stable angina and single vessel disease treated with PTCA obtain greater symptom relief than those treated medically (Parisi et al., 1992). However, the procedure has an associated higher risk of MI and emergency CABG. Patients with stable angina treated by CABG obtain greater early (first 3 months) symptom relief than those treated by PTCA but each mode of treatment has equal risk of cardiac death and non-fatal MI after almost 3 years (RITA Trial Participants, 1993). In addition, cost consideration and limited availability of invasive angiogram facilities suggest a greater cost-benefit yield from secondary prevention measures. When PTCA is carried out in MI where thrombolysis is contraindicated, the benefit may be particularly evident in patients with anterior MI, over 65 years old and with persistent tachycardia (Grines et al., 1993; Zijlstra et al., 1993; Gibbons et al., 1993).

Patients with persisting anginal pain and ECG changes suggestive of non-reperfusion, those with contra-indications to thrombolysis and patients in cardiogenic shock may be considered for either primary or bail-out PTCA. Procedural success rates are good but survival to discharge rates in such patients with cardiogenic shock are poor.

INTRACORONARY STENTS

In trials comparing the use of stents with PTCA, the deployment of stents is associated with higher procedural success rates and lower restenosis rates. Experience with the use of stent deployment in emergencies arising from coronary occlusion or dissection is growing. Inhibitors of platelet activation such as ticlopidine and other specific glycoprotein IIb/IIIa receptor inhibitors have reduced the incidence of stent thrombosis but increase the risk of bleeding complications while ticlopidine is infrequently associated with neurtopenia. Various regimens are employed including the use of ticlopidine before elective stenting, four weeks of therapy after the procedure and with special attention to neutrophil counts.

CORONARY ARTERY BYPASS GRAFTING

Indications for emergency surgery in the early post-MI setting include:

- Failed PTCA with persistent pain or haemodynamic compromise.
- Papillary muscle rupture.
- Ventricular septal defect or rupture of the free wall.
- Acute mitral regurgitation with severe heart failure.
- Left main stem stenosis and severe three vessel disease with poor LV function/unstable angina.

TEMPORARY PACING IN MYOCARDIAL INFARCTION

Temporary pacing (See appendix C) is warranted in refractory bradyarrhythmias, and is sometimes useful in tachyarrhythmias when under or overdrive pacing can be used to terminate an SVT. Transcutaneous pacing may be useful while awaiting transvenous pacing. The femoral transvenous route is probably the easiest but, in the absence of fluoroscopy, the internal jugular vein allows a more direct entry to the right ventricle. Alternatively, the subclavian vein may be used. The indications for temporary pacing in acute MI are:

- Sinus or junctional bradycardia associated with syncope, hypotension or heart failure unresponsive to atropine.
- Second degree (Figure 18c) and complete heart block (Figure 18d) in anterior MI; in inferior MI if there is haemodynamic compromise.
- Recent onset right bundle branch block with either left or right axis deviation, alternating left and right bundle branch block and second degree heart block associated with an anterior infarct.
- Complete heart block, in anterior infarcts and unstable inferior MI.
- Episodes of asystole.

ANTITACHYCARDIA PACING

Overdrive or underdrive pacing may be employed to terminate a tachyarrhythmia. To carry this out, insert a temporary pacing lead and pace at a rate 20–30% faster than the patient's rate for a short time interval (30–60 seconds). Similarly, underdrive pacing involves fixed pacing at a rate slower than the tachycardia rate.

HAEMODYNAMIC MONITORING

The insertion of a Swan Ganz catheter allows the evaluation of right atrial, right ventricular, pulmonary artery, and indirect left atrial (pulmonary capillary wedge) pressures (Figure 23), as well as cardiac output. This requires considerable operator experience and may be carried out in cardiogenic shock or moderate to severe left ventricular failure. It is important to avoid inflating the balloon in the pulmonary capillary for more than 15 seconds at a time. Hourly heparin flushes are required to prevent clot formation at the tip of the cathether and the catheter itself should not be left in for more than 3 days because of the risk of infection.

HAEMODYNAMIC MONITORING

	PCWP/PADP (mmHg)	ARTERIAL PRESSURE (mmHg)	CARDIAC OUTPUT (L/min)	THERAPY
Normal	< 15	> 100/60	3.5 - 5.0	
Acute pul. oedema	>25	Normal	Low	Nitrates
Cardiogenic shock	Variable Usually high	Low	Low	Dobutamine +/–Dopamine
Acute pul. oedema+shock	> 25	Low	Low	Dobutamine +Nitrates
Hypovolaemia	< 15	Low	Normal	Replace fluid

PRESSURE TRACINGS IN HAEMODYNAMIC MONITORING

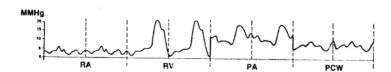

RA = right atrium
RV = right ventricle
PA = pulmonary artery
PCW = pulmonary capillary wedge
PADP = pulmonary artery diastolic pressure

Figure 23 Intra-cardiac pressures detected by haemodynamic monitoring.

9

INVESTIGATIONS POST-MYOCARDIAL INFARCTION

EXERCISE ECG TEST.

In fully mobile post-infarction patients an exercise ECG should be carried out at day 7–10. Positive tests at low work loads suggest a poorer prognosis and may be an indication for early angiography. Contraindications to stress testing in the post-MI period are:

- Unstable angina.
- Suspected left main stem disease.
- Cardiac failure.
- Complete heart block.
- Severe aortic stenosis.
- Suspected aortic dissection.

Reported mortality rates are ~ 1:10 000.

ECHOCARDIOGRAPHY

Bedside echocardiography (if available) in the early the stages of atypical chest pain and non-diagnostic ECG changes may help to exclude pericardial effusion. Similarly, an estimate of infarct size, chamber size, LV and valve function can be made at an early stage. The aortic root can also be visualized and an assessment of root size can be made. Transoesophageal echocardiography (TOE) is probably the bedside investigation of choice in excluding aortic dissection.

NUCLEAR CARDIOLOGY IMAGING

In experienced hands, nuclear scanning of the myocardium using dipyridamole or exercise thallium scanning allows precise definition of the extent, distribution and reversibility of ischaemia. However, there is a significant incidence of false positive tests especially in females. False negative imaging is a relatively rare phonemenon.

24-HOUR AMBULATORY ECG MONITORING

Ambulatory ECG monitoring allows for the prognostic assessment of patients who have sustained moderate to severe LV damage. Patients exhibiting recurrent sustained ventricular rhythms on ambulation have poorer prognosis long term.

CORONARY ANGIOGRAPHY

In the stable post-MI patient, coronary angiography is carried out for the prognostic assessment of coronary artery disease and left ventricular function. On the basis of symptoms and the extent of disease demonstrated on angiography, a therapeutic plan can be devised and continued medical management or bypass surgery may be warranted. Assuming proper patient evaluation before this invasive procedure, the associated risks, e.g. stroke, are small – of the order of 1 per 1000 tests. It may also be required in subjects whose pain fails to settle in the post-infarction period, in subjects with subendocardial infarction who are at risk of subsequent transmural infarction, those with positive exercise tests at low work loads/with symptoms or those who have a high risk occupation, e.g. construction workers, public transport vehicle drivers, etc.

10

CARDIAC REHABILITATION AND SECONDARY PREVENTION

IMMEDIATE MEASURES

The aim of cardiac rehabilitation is to return the patient to a normal lifestyle. A meta-analysis of studies has shown a benefit from rehabilitation equal to that from either thrombolysis, aspirin or ACE inhibitors (See **EBM note** below). Cardiac rehabilitation can begin immediately in the CCU with leg, arm and breathing exercises performed in bed. Where possible, the cardiac rehabilitation nurse introduces the patient to the basic concepts of rehabilitation inviting questions, allaying anxiety and ultimately inviting the patient to attend the formal rehabilitation course after the present illness. At this early stage it is often necessary to reiterate basic information repeatedly to provide the necessary reassurance as anxiety and fatigue both impair the patient's attention span. This information and reassurance can be provided in many ways:

- Speak slowly and clearly to patient, spouse and family members who themselves need to be informed in order to avoid an overly protective attitude.
- Use information booklets to provide basic information
- Use cardiac rehabilitation video or audio-tapes
- Encourage the patient to visit the cardiac rehabilitation gym (where available) to witness other patients overcoming similar difficulties.

▶ Specific Issues Often Raised by Patients

Driving
Not adviseable for about 6 weeks post MI and not if it provokes angina. Patients with proven infarction are likely to lose their HGV or Public Service Licence although they may still drive a car. In some countries (UK) it is a legal requirement to inform the licensing authority that he or

she has suffered a myocardial infarction. In the Republic of Ireland, the decision as to whether the patient may drive a car again rests with the physician.

Sexual activity

Patients are often reluctant to discuss sexual activity. If possible, an opportunity should be allowed for this matter to be discussed on a one to one basis. In general, sexual activity should be treated like any other form of physical activity, starting gradually a week or two following discharge from hospital.

Exercise

A programme designed to suit the patient should be discussed. This varies according to the patient's previous level of fitness and expectations. Essentially, the exercise can be as vigorous as one likes but aerobic, i.e. low intensity and long distance fitness is of greater benefit to the heart.

Return to work

Can take place within a matter of weeks of the infarct depending on the job involved and the individual's expectations. Sometimes it is necessary to liaise with the patient's employer and social worker to relocate within the work place.

EBM note: A meta-analysis of trials of the efficacy of various cardiac rehabilitation programmes (O'Connor et al. 1989) has shown that a benefit of the order of 20% mortality reduction is attainable with cardiac rehabilitation. Given that patients are screened before commencing a particular programme, this selection bias could have a significant bearing on the outcome of the trial. In addition, publication bias, where only trials showing a positive outcome are published could significantly influence an overview of such trials.

▶ Mobilisation

Patients who are pain free and haemodynamically stable may sit out within 12 hours of the cessation of pain. Within a further 24–48 hours, they may be transferred to the general ward/recovery area to increase their independence and mobility aiming to be fully ambulant at one week after MI. Look to the long-term and establish exercise goals which are realistic and take account of the patient's social circumstances and previous level of fitness. Perhaps a mile a day at the end of the first week home, two miles at the end of the second and 21 miles a week thereafter is reasonable. Define a target date for return to work if appropriate to give encouragement.

▶ Total Risk Evaluation

Physical exercise is important for both physical fitness and confidence, but forms only one part of secondary prevention. Cardiovascular risk factors interact to increase *total risk* and all need to be considered in designing a programme to minimise risk (Appendix E).

ACTIONS TO REDUCE TOTAL RISK

- Smoking: The physician's firm, sympathetic but explicit advice is probably the single most effective anti-smoking measure. Patients should be advised that those who continue to smoke have twice the death rate of those who stop and that no drug is as effective.
- Hypertension: Decide on long-term treatment; look for end-organ damage and aim for a blood pressure of less than 140/ 90 for most subjects.
- Hyperlipidaemia: It is now accepted that reduction of serum total and LDL cholesterol reduces progression of coronary disease, may induce regression, and reduces risk of further cardiac events in patients who have established coronary heart disease with high (4S study) and average (CARE study) serum total cholesterol levels, as well those with high cholesterol levels at risk of developing such disease (WOS-COP study). This reduction can be achieved by dietary advice instituted for a finite (3–6 months) period and where necessary, by medication after this period has elapsed. The decision to institute such therapies should be taken as early as possible but should be based on an evaluation of total risk (See Appendix E and *Recommendations of the Task Force of the ESC/EAS/ESH*, Appendix F). Check the full lipid profile within 24 hours of admission. Aim for a total cholesterol of 5mmol/L in most subjects, using a medication such as a statin as required.
- Diabetes: Diabetes increases threefold the risk of cardiovascular disease. Good glucose control limits microvascular complications. Dietary restriction, weight control, the addition of oral hypoglycaemic agents and if necessary, insulin each helps to attain this goal. Look for proteinuria, glycosuria, neuropathy, retinopathy and evidence of peripheral vascular disease. Aim for a fasting glucose of less than 7mmol/L and a post prandial glucose of less than 10mmol/L.

Other advice on individual social circumstances, employment and stress management problems may also be required.

● Features of the infarction itself or pertaining to the patient's risk factor profile may aid risk stratification:

> Anterior MI/Inferior MI?
> Thrombolysis given?
> Poor exercise tolerance on stress testing?
> Easily inducible angina and ECG changes on stress testing?
> Adverse risk factor profile?
> Severe coronary artery disease at angiography?
> Left ventricular dysfunction/hypertrophy

● Check the medications and the patient's familiarity with them. Minimise and simplify the regimen.

GTN spray sl is useful in infrequent stable post infarction angina.
Oral nitrates are used prophylactically in more frequent angina
Aspirin improves both short and long term prognosis.
ACE inhibitors, instituted early, reduce mortality after MI in those with impaired LV function.
Beta-antagonists improve prognosis in high risk subjects
Anticoagulants for those with LV aneurysm or dysrhythmias which increase risk of embolism.

EBM note: In the UK ASPIRE study, 20% of patients with AMI, PTCA, CABG, and acute myocardial ischaemia were still smoking at 6 months after the procedure or event. Up to one quarter remained hypertensive. Over 75% had a serum total cholesterol greater than 5.2mmol/L. One fifth were not taking aspirin. One third were taking a betablocker and one quarter were taking an ACE inhibitor. Trials of the efficacy of ACE inhibition instituted in the early phase post-infarction also suggest that a benefit of the order of 20% reduced mortality can be achieved (Kober et al. 1995).

Appendix A

Commonly used drugs

INTRAVENOUS ADMINISTRATION OF DRUGS

Isoprenaline (Saventrine 2mg/2ml)
Route of administration: iv infusion only.
Usual dose range: 0.5 μg/min–10μg/min.
2mg added to 500ml of glucose 5% results in a solution containing 4μg/ml of isoprenaline, (see table for corresponding doses).

Dose of isoprenaline

µg/min	mls/hr
0.5	7.5
1.0	15.0
2.0	30.0
4.0	60.0
6.0	90.0
8.0	120.0
10.0	150.0

Verapamil (Isoptin 5mg/2ml)
Routes of administration: slow iv injection.
Dilute a 2ml amp(5mg) to 5ml water for injection or normal saline 0.9% giving a resultant solution of 1 mg/ml. This should be given slowly over at least two minutes under close monitoring of ECG and blood pressure.

▶ Thombolytic therapy

i. Streptokinase
Reconstitute using 5ml normal saline and dilute to the desired final volume (usually 50–100ml) with normal saline, glucose 5% w/v or Hartmann's solution. Give 1.5 million unit dose in an infusion over 60 mins.

ii. t-PA

Reconstitute each 50mg vial in 50ml of water for injection provided. This results in a 1 mg/ml solution.

A total dose of 100mg should be given intravenously over 3hrs as follows:

10% of the total dose as an iv bolus over 1–2 mins.

50% of the total dose as an infusion over 1 hour.

40% of the total dose as an infusion over the subsequent 2 hours.

Patients weighing less than 67kg should receive a total dose of 1.5mg/kg according to the above schedule.

The accelerated regimen of t-PA is:

Give bolus of 15mg (15ml of solvent.) iv stat.

Then infuse 50ml over 30mins (0.75ml/kg) followed by 35ml over 60mins (0.5ml/kg).

Adrenaline infusion table

Dilute 3mg of adrenaline (1mg/ml inj) to 50ml, giving a final concentration of $60\mu g$/ml.

Dose μg/min	Infusion Rate ml/hr
1	1
2	2
3	3
4	4
5	5
6	6
7	7
8	8
9	9
10	10

Adrenaline is compatible with glucose 5% and normal saline.
* To be administered via syringe pump.

Dose chart for dobutamine

Patient weight (kg)

Infusion rate [ml/hr] for a solution of dobutamine 250mg/50ml

Dose µg/kg/min	40	45	50	55	60	65	70	75	80	85	90	95	100
1	0.5	0.5	0.6	0.7	0.7	0.8	0.8	0.9	1.0	1.0	1.1	1.1	1.2
2	1.0	1.1	1.2	1.3	1.4	1.6	1.7	1.8	1.9	2.0	2.2	2.3	2.4
3	1.4	1.6	1.8	2.0	2.2	2.3	2.5	2.7	2.9	3.1	3.2	3.4	3.6
4	1.9	2.2	2.4	2.6	2.9	3.1	3.4	3.6	3.8	4.1	4.3	4.6	4.8
5	2.4	2.7	3.0	3.3	3.6	3.9	4.2	4.5	4.8	5.1	5.4	5.7	6.0
6	2.9	3.2	3.6	4.0	4.3	4.7	5.0	5.4	5.8	6.1	6.5	6.8	7.2
7	3.4	3.8	4.2	4.6	5.0	5.5	5.9	6.3	6.7	7.1	7.6	8.0	8.4
8	3.8	4.3	4.8	5.3	5.8	6.2	6.7	7.2	7.7	8.2	8.6	9.1	9.6
9	4.3	4.9	5.4	5.9	6.5	7.0	7.6	8.1	8.6	9.2	9.7	10.3	10.8
10	4.8	5.4	6.0	6.6	7.2	7.8	8.4	9.0	9.6	10.2	10.8	11.4	12.0
11	5.3	5.9	6.6	7.3	7.9	8.6	9.2	9.9	10.6	11.2	11.9	12.5	13.2
12	5.8	6.5	7.2	7.9	8.6	9.4	10.1	10.8	11.5	12.2	13.0	13.7	14.4
13	6.2	7.0	7.8	8.6	9.4	10.1	10.9	11.7	12.5	13.3	14.0	14.8	15.6
14	6.7	7.6	8.4	9.2	10.1	10.9	11.8	12.6	13.4	14.3	15.1	16.0	16.8
15	7.2	8.1	9.0	9.9	10.8	11.7	12.6	13.5	14.4	15.3	16.2	17.1	18.0
16	7.7	8.6	9.6	10.6	11.5	12.5	13.4	14.4	15.4	16.3	17.3	18.2	19.2
17	8.2	9.2	10.2	11.2	12.2	13.3	14.3	15.3	16.3	17.3	18.4	19.4	20.4
18	8.6	9.7	10.8	11.9	13.0	14.0	15.1	16.2	17.3	18.4	19.4	20.5	21.6
19	9.1	10.3	11.4	12.5	13.7	14.8	16.0	17.1	18.2	19.4	20.5	21.7	22.8
20	9.6	10.8	12.0	13.2	14.4	15.6	16.8	18.0	19.2	20.4	21.6	22.8	24.0

* To be administered via syringe pump.

Dose chart for dopexamine for peripheral administration (50mg/50ml)

Dose µg/kg/min	Patient weight (kg)												
	40	45	50	55	60	65	70	75	80	85	90	95	100
	Infusion rate [ml/hr] for a solution of dopexamine 50mg/50ml												
0.5	1.2	1.4	1.5	1.7	1.8	2.0	2.1	2.3	2.4	2.6	2.7	2.9	3.0
1.0	2.4	2.7	3.0	3.3	3.6	3.9	4.2	4.5	4.8	5.1	5.4	5.7	6.0
1.5	3.6	4.1	4.5	5.0	5.4	5.9	6.3	6.8	7.2	7.7	8.1	8.6	9.0
2.0	4.8	5.4	6.0	6.6	7.2	7.8	8.4	9.0	9.6	10.2	10.8	11.4	12.0
2.5	6.0	6.8	7.5	8.3	9.0	9.8	10.5	11.3	12.0	12.8	13.5	14.3	15.0
3.0	7.2	8.1	9.0	9.9	10.8	11.7	12.6	13.5	14.4	15.3	16.2	17.1	18.0
3.5	8.4	9.4	10.5	11.6	12.6	13.7	14.7	15.8	16.8	17.9	18.9	20.0	21.0
4.0	9.6	10.8	12.0	13.2	14.4	15.6	16.8	18.0	19.2	20.4	21.6	22.8	24.0
4.5	10.8	12.2	13.5	14.9	16.2	17.6	18.9	20.3	21.6	23.0	24.3	25.7	27.0
5.0	12.0	13.5	15.0	16.5	18.0	19.5	21.0	22.5	24.0	25.5	27.0	28.5	30.0
5.5	13.2	14.9	16.5	18.2	19.8	21.5	23.1	24.8	26.4	28.1	29.7	31.4	33.0
6.0	14.2	16.2	18.0	19.8	21.6	23.4	25.2	27.0	28.8	30.6	32.4	34.2	36.0

Dopexamine may be diluted with normal saline or glucose 5%
* To be administered via syringe pump.

Dose chart for dopexamine for central line use (100mg/50ml)

Patient weight (kg)

Infusion rate [ml/hr] for a solution of dopexamine 100mg/50ml

Dose µg/kg/min	40	45	50	55	60	65	70	75	80	85	90	95	100
0.5	0.6	0.7	0.8	0.8	0.9	1.0	1.1	1.1	1.2	1.3	1.4	1.4	1.5
1.0	1.2	1.4	1.5	1.7	1.8	2.0	2.1	2.3	2.4	2.6	2.7	2.9	3.0
1.5	1.8	2.0	2.3	2.5	2.7	2.9	3.2	3.4	3.6	3.8	4.1	4.3	4.5
2.0	2.4	2.7	3.0	3.3	3.6	3.9	4.2	4.5	4.8	5.1	5.4	5.7	6.0
2.5	3.0	3.4	3.8	4.1	4.5	4.9	5.3	5.6	6.0	6.4	6.8	7.1	7.5
3.0	3.6	4.1	4.5	5.0	5.4	5.9	6.3	6.8	7.2	7.7	8.1	8.6	9.0
3.5	4.2	4.7	5.3	5.8	6.3	6.8	7.4	7.9	8.4	8.9	9.4	10.0	10.5
4.0	4.8	5.4	6.0	6.6	7.2	7.8	8.4	9.0	9.6	10.2	10.8	11.4	12.0
4.5	5.4	6.1	6.8	7.4	8.1	8.8	9.4	10.1	10.8	11.5	12.2	12.8	13.5
5.0	6.0	6.8	7.5	8.3	9.0	9.8	10.5	11.3	12.0	12.8	13.5	14.3	15.0
5.5	6.6	7.4	8.3	9.1	9.9	10.7	11.6	12.4	13.2	14.0	14.9	15.7	16.5
6.0	7.2	8.2	9.0	10.0	10.8	11.8	12.6	13.6	14.4	15.4	16.2	17.2	18.0

Dopexamine may be diluted with normal saline or glucose 5%
* To be administered via syringe pump.

Dose chart for dopamine infusion in fluid restriction

Dose µg/kg/min	Patient weight (kg)												
	40	45	50	55	60	65	70	75	80	85	90	95	100
	Infusion rate [ml/hr] for a solution of dopamine 200mg/50ml												
1	0.6	0.7	0.8	0.8	0.9	1.0	1.1	1.1	1.2	1.3	1.4	1.4	1.5
2	1.2	1.4	1.5	1.7	1.8	2.0	2.1	2.3	2.4	2.6	2.7	2.9	3.0
2.5	1.5	1.7	1.9	2.1	2.3	2.4	2.6	2.8	3.0	3.2	3.4	3.6	3.8
3	1.8	2.0	2.3	2.5	2.7	2.9	3.2	3.4	3.6	3.8	4.1	4.3	4.5
4	2.4	2.7	3.0	3.3	3.6	3.9	4.2	4.5	4.8	5.1	5.4	5.7	6.0
5	3.0	3.4	3.8	4.1	4.5	4.9	5.3	5.6	6.0	6.4	6.8	7.1	7.5
10	6.0	6.8	7.5	8.3	9.0	9.8	10.5	11.3	12.0	12.8	13.5	14.3	15.0
11	6.6	7.4	8.3	9.1	9.9	10.7	11.6	12.4	13.2	14.0	14.9	15.7	16.5
12	7.2	8.1	9.0	9.9	10.8	11.7	12.6	13.5	14.4	15.3	16.2	17.1	18.0
13	7.8	8.8	9.8	10.7	11.7	12.7	13.7	14.6	15.6	16.6	17.6	18.5	19.5
14	8.4	9.4	10.5	11.6	12.6	13.7	14.7	15.8	16.8	17.9	18.9	20.0	21.0
15	9.0	10.1	11.3	12.4	13.5	14.6	15.8	16.9	18.0	19.1	20.3	21.4	22.5
16	9.6	10.8	12.0	13.2	14.4	15.6	16.8	18.0	19.2	20.4	21.6	22.8	24.0
17	10.2	11.5	12.8	14.0	15.3	16.6	17.9	19.1	20.4	21.7	23.0	24.2	25.5
18	10.8	12.2	13.5	14.9	16.2	17.6	18.9	20.3	21.6	23.0	24.3	25.7	27.0
19	11.4	12.8	14.3	15.7	17.1	18.5	20.0	21.4	22.8	24.2	25.7	27.1	28.5
20	12.0	13.5	15.0	16.5	18.0	19.5	21.0	22.5	24.0	25.5	27.0	28.5	30.0

* To be administered via syringe pump.

Dose chart for dopamine infusion

Dose µg/kg/min	Patient weight (kg)												
	40	45	50	55	60	65	70	75	80	85	90	95	100
	Infusion rate [ml/hr] for a solution dopamine 400mg/250ml												
5.0	7.5	8.4	9.4	10.3	11.3	12.2	13.1	14.1	15.0	15.9	16.9	17.8	18.8
7.0	10.5	11.8	13.1	14.4	15.8	17.1	18.4	19.7	21.0	22.3	23.6	24.9	26.3
9.0	13.5	15.2	16.9	18.6	20.3	21.9	23.6	25.3	27.0	28.7	30.4	32.1	33.8
10.0	15.0	16.9	18.8	20.6	22.5	24.4	26.3	28.1	30.0	31.9	33.8	35.6	37.5
11.0	16.5	18.6	20.6	22.7	24.8	26.8	28.9	30.9	33.0	35.1	37.1	39.2	41.3
13.0	19.5	21.9	24.4	26.8	29.3	31.7	34.1	36.6	39.0	41.4	43.9	46.3	48.8
15.0	22.5	25.3	28.1	30.9	33.8	36.6	39.4	42.2	45.0	47.8	50.6	53.4	56.3
17.0	25.5	28.7	31.9	35.1	38.3	41.4	44.6	47.8	51.0	54.2	57.4	60.6	63.8
19.0	28.5	32.1	35.6	39.2	42.8	46.3	49.9	53.4	57.0	60.6	64.1	67.7	71.3
20.0	30.0	33.8	37.5	41.3	45.0	48.8	52.5	56.3	60.0	63.8	67.5	71.3	75.0

Dopamine may be added to glucose 5% or normal saline
* To be administered via volumetric pump.

Dose chart for dopamine ***Renal regimen***

Infusion rate [ml/hr] for a solution of dopamine 200mg/250ml

Dose µg/kg/min	Patient weight (kg)												
	40	45	50	55	60	65	70	75	80	85	90	95	100
1.0	3.0	3.4	3.8	4.1	4.5	4.9	5.3	5.6	6.0	6.4	6.8	7.1	7.5
3.0	6.0	6.8	7.5	8.3	9.0	9.8	10.5	11.3	12.0	12.8	13.5	14.3	15.0
2.0	9.0	10.1	11.3	12.4	13.5	14.6	15.8	16.9	18.0	19.1	20.3	21.4	22.5
4.0	12.0	13.5	15.0	16.5	18.0	19.5	21.0	22.5	24.0	25.5	27.0	28.5	30.0
5.0	15.0	16.9	18.8	20.6	22.5	24.4	26.3	28.1	30.0	31.9	33.8	35.6	37.5

Dopamine may be added to glucose 5% or normal saline
* To be administered via volumetric pump.

Glyceryl trinitrate infusion table

Dilute glyceryl trinitrate amps 25mg/5ml to 50ml, giving a final concentration of 500μg/ml. Glyceryl trinitrate is incompatible with PVC and should be administered using non-PVC containers and giving sets, e.g. syringe driver and Lecto-spiral giving set (Vygon).

The following table gives the dose of glyceryl trinitrate in microgrammes per minute for a preset infusion rate in ml/hour.

Dose μg/min	Infusion Rate ml/hr	Dose μg/min	Infusion Rate ml/hr
8.3	1.0	25.0	3.0
12.5	1.5	29.2	3.5
13.3	1.6	33.3	4.0
14.1	1.7	37.5	4.5
15.0	1.8	41.7	5.0
15.8	1.9	45.8	5.5
16.6	2.0	50.0	6.0
17.5	2.1	54.2	6.5
18.3	2.2	58.3	7.0
19.1	2.3	62.5	7.5
20.0	2.4	66.7	8.0
21.6	2.6	70.8	8.5
22.5	2.7	75.0	9.0
23.3	2.8	79.0	9.5
24.2	2.9	83.0	10.0

Glyceryl trinitrate is compatible with glucose 5% and normal saline.

CARDIOPULMONARY RESUSCITATION PROTOCOLS

▶ Cardiac arrest

Cardiac arrest has occurred when there is:
1. loss of consciousness
2. absent femoral or carotid pulse
3. no spontaneous respiration
Irreversible brain damage may occur if CPR is not started within 3 minutes.

MANAGEMENT
If monitor shows ventricular fibrillation and a defibrillator is immediately available, defibrillate first. In all other situations the establishment of a clear airway, effective ventilation and external cardiac massage have absolute precedence and should not be delayed.

▶ Basic cardiopulmonary resuscitation

1. Determine unresponsiveness and call out for help:
   Gently shake shoulder
   Shout 'Are you OK'
   Call out and activate the emergency service
2. Open airway by a combined movement of head tilt and chin lift:
   In suspected neck injuries, the jaw thrust method should be used. Any obvious obstruction, e.g. broken or displaced dentures, solid material is removed with a finger sweep. Suction if liquid present.
3. Check for breathing:
   Look for chest movements,
   Listen for breath sounds
   Feel for exhaled air at the back of the hand
   If not breathing, artificial ventilation should be initiated.
   Mouth to mask: Ensure tight seal. Initially, give two slow expired breaths of air, each sufficient to cause the chest to rise. Allow for

expirations between ventilations. Each breath should last 1–1.5 seconds. If chest not expanding, check and reopen airway.

Ambubag/mask preferable (when available): Open airway, insert oral airway and apply mask. If difficult to hold, use both hands to maintain open airway and ensure tight seal whilst another person provides ventilation using Ambubag.

4. Check circulation: determine pulselessness by palpating carotid pulse on near side (other hand on forehead to maintain head tilt).

Closed chest compression will circulate blood to vital organs (less than 25% (max.) of normal cardiac output), by increasing intra-thoracic pressure during the compressions. Subjects should be placed on a firm surface, and effective chest compression should produce a palpable carotid/femoral pulse.

Proper rescuer position is necessary. Kneel beside the subject, with the heel of the hand two finger widths from the lower end of the sternum, depress the sternum 1.5–2 inches each time, keeping arms straight and shoulder directly above hands. Fingers are kept off the chest. For one-person CPR, the compression: ventilation ratio is 15:2; chest compression rate is 80/min. Check for the return of pulse and spontaneous respiration after 4 cycles. If none, resume with two ventilations followed by compressions.

At entry of a second rescuer: Second rescuer checks carotid/femoral pulse for effective compressions and calls out 'STOP' to check for spontaneous breathing and pulse. Second rescuer ventilates once, states 'NO pulse, continue CPR'. First rescuer resumes cardiac compressions. For two-person CPR the compression: ventilation ratio is 5:1; chest compression rate is 80/min.

▶ Advanced Cardiac Life Support (ACLS)

The algorithm shown comprises the actions which should be taken in pulseless VT/VF, asystole, and electromechanical dissociation or pulse-less electrical activity. Defibrillation paddles may be used to read the underlying rhythm and appropriate action is then quickly taken once the rhythm is interpreted. The ACLS team leader should ensure that a member of the team establishes adequate ventilation by intubation as soon as possible (but not before initial defibrillation in pulseless VT/VF). Access to a large peripheral vein (preferably antecubital) is also important to allow delivery of medication. Adrenaline, lignocaine, atropine and bretylium, at 2–2.5 times the iv dose and diluted to a 10ml

ADVANCED CARDIAC LIFE SUPPORT

Responsive? No → **Breathing?** No → **Pulse?** No → **Start CPR** 2:15

☎ **Call for help**
Including
- defibrillator
- airway adjuncts
- oxygen
- emergency kit

Consider 2 rescuer CPR
1:5
and
mouth-to-mask ventilation

Precordial thump

Place paddles correctly

If flat trace, check switches, connections and gain.

Give oxygen

Intubate

Cannulate large vein

Continue CPR

EMD
QRS without palpable pulse

Think of, and if indicated, give specific treatment for:

- hypovolaemia
- tension pneumothorax
- cardiac tamponade
- pulmonary embolism
- drug overdose/intoxication
- hypothermia
- electrolyte imbalance

If not already
- intubate
- iv access

Adrenaline 1mg iv

10 CPR sequences of 5:1 compression/ventilation

Consider
- pressor agents
- calcium
- alkalising agents
- adrenaline 5 mg iv

VF
PULSELESS VT

Precordial thump

DC shock 200 J 1
DC shock 200 J 2
DC shock 360 J 3

If not already
- intubate
- iv access

Adrenaline 1mg iv

10 CPR sequences of 5:1 compression/ventilation

DC shock 360 J 4
DC shock 360 J 5
DC shock 360 J 6

Notes:
I   The interval between shocks 3 and 4 should not be > 2 mins
II Adrenaline given during loop approx every 2-3 mins
III Continue loops for as long as defibrillation is indicated
IV After 3 loops consider - alkalising agents
    - antiarrhythmic agents

ASYSTOLE

Precordial thump

VF excluded? → yes
no

DC shock 200 J
DC shock 200 J
DC shock 360 J

If not already
- intubate
- iv access

Adrenaline 1mg iv

10 CPR sequences of 5:1 compression/ventilation

(Atropine 3 mg iv once only)

Electrical activity evident? → no
yes
Pace

Note:
If no response after 3 cycles consider high dose adrenaline 5 mg iv

---

If an IV line cannot be established, consider giving double or triple doses of adrenaline or atropine via an endotracheal tube.

PROLONGED RESUSCITATION:
Consider alkalising agents, e.g. 50 mmol sodium bicarbonate (50ml of 8.4%) or according to blood gas results.

POST RESUSCITATION CARE
Check
- arterial blood gases
- electrolytes
- chest x-ray
Observe monitor and treat patient in an intensive care area.

European Resuscitation Council

volume with normal saline, may be given down the ET tube via a long catheter if iv access is impossible. Ventilation should immediately follow to distribute the drug.

● In pulseless VT/VF, the emphasis is on early defibrillation, appropriate use of antidysrhythmic agents and later (if at all) use of alkalizing agents, e.g consider after three loops of the algorhythm. In specific circumstances, however, alkalizing agents may be given, namely acidosis, hyperkalemia, and tricyclic or barbiturate overdose. Deliver the first shocks as three consecutive discharges of 200J, 200J and 360J. Do not allow basic life support to interrupt the sequence of the shocks unless there is undue delay with the charging of the defibrillator. Check the rhythm after each discharge and the pulse after all three shocks. Once the first three shocks have been delivered and, assuming they are unsuccessful, achieve rapid intubation and ventilate with 100% oxygen, administer appropriate drugs, continue chest compressions and deliver 360J shocks as appropriate.

● In asystole and electromechanical dissociation-pulseless electrical activity early consideration should be given to possible underlying causes some of which are remediable. If asystole is seen on the monitor **always** check a second lead before taking action. Do not shock in asystole. Atropine is given in a dose (3mg) which is vagolytic. Consider pacing.

Prognosis
Primary VF frequently responds to prompt defibrillation. Secondary ventricular fibrillation, i.e. VF and asystole in the presence of major medical complications are less amenable to resuscitation. Outlook in electromechanical dissociation depends on the aetiology. Profound bradycardia not infrequently progresses to asystole.

When to stop resuscitation
In most cases, resuscitation attempts may be stopped after 30 minutes if there is refractory asystole or electromechanical dissociation. These primary dysrhythmias have a poorer prognosis than primary VF/VT. Prolonged efforts are worthwhile in young people, hypothermia, electrocution, poisoning and drowning. The ultimate decision as to when to stop should rest with the person in charge of the CPR.

American heart association guidelines on temporary pacing

▶ Class 1 (recommended):
Symptomatic bradycardia
3rd degree AV block
2nd degree Mobitz 2 block
also, new onset LBBB
RBBB with hemiblock

▶ Class 2a (likely useful):
2nd degree Mobitz 1
Sinus pauses (with symptoms)
VT overdrive

▶ Class 2b Role? (possibly useful): in special circumstances
1st degree AV block with symptomatic bradycardia
Presenting BBB with symptomatic bradycardia

▶ Class 3 (not indicated):
1st degree AV block
Stable 2nd degree Mobitz 1
Idioventricular rhythm (slow VT)

Appendix D

Interesting ECGs

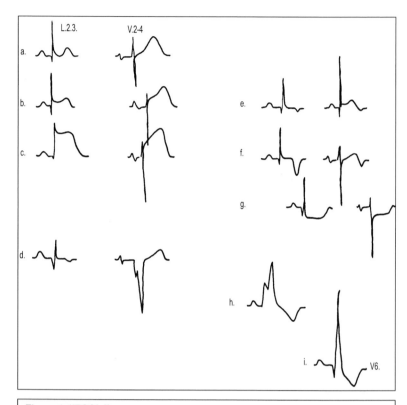

Figure 1 "ECG's"

(a) Normal: the record is often normal in angina pectoris and in the early stages of infarction.

(b) Early(1–6 hours): ST elevation. The ST segment is often elevated > 1mm in the standard leads and more than 2mm in the V leads. Where there is overlap between normality and early abnormality, check serial recordings (every 20–30 minutes) and cardiac enzymes.

(c) Classic infarction patterns: these may take 1–6 hours to evolve.

(d) Old infarction: inferior MI: L2, 3, AVF; anterior MI: V2–4–6.

(e) Minor non-specific changes may be suspicious in the context of cardiac pain.

(f) Non-specific ST-T changes are highly suspicious in the context of cardiac chest pain.

(g) Diffuse ST depression: likely subendocardial ischaemia/infarction if cardiac pain is present.

(h) Left bundle branch block: typically dominates the record and is usually abnormal. If present in the context of cardiac pain, anterior infarction is likely.

(i) LV strain pattern: not necessarily a marker of ischaemia, it may occur in the presence of aortic stenosis or hypertensive heart disease. Check serial cardiac enzymes.

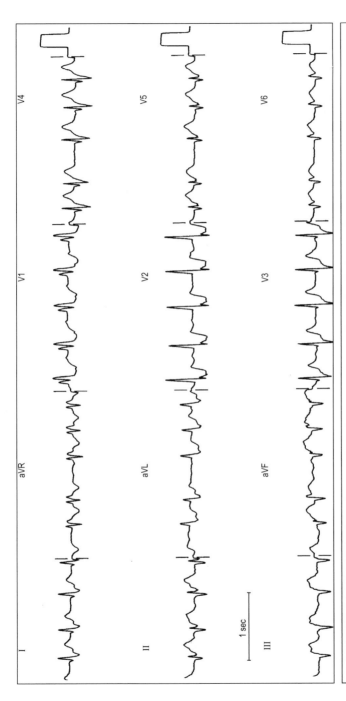

Figure 2 Old inferior infarction

Atrial fibrillation with rate of 100–140 per minute is noted; right bundle branch block (see V1). Q wave noted with poor R wave in lead L2, 3, AVF, V5, V6.

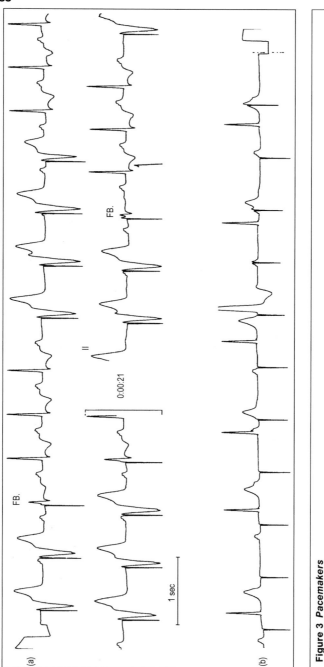

Figure 3 Pacemakers

(a) Pacing (ventricular) rhythm with rate 70/ minute; sinus rhythm with PR-interval 0.25 sec when the pacemaker is inhibited. The third beat is a fusion beat denoted as FB.

(b) Pacing spike with no capture. Sino-atrial block with nodal escape rhythm and rate of 36/minute evident.

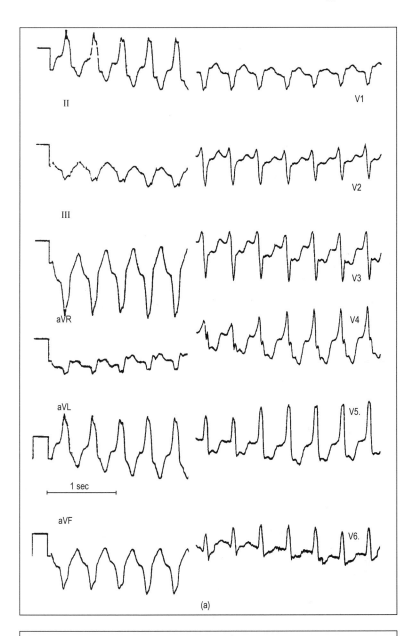

(a)

Figure 4(a) *Ventricular tachycardia*
Ventricular tachycardia with left bundle branch block configuration

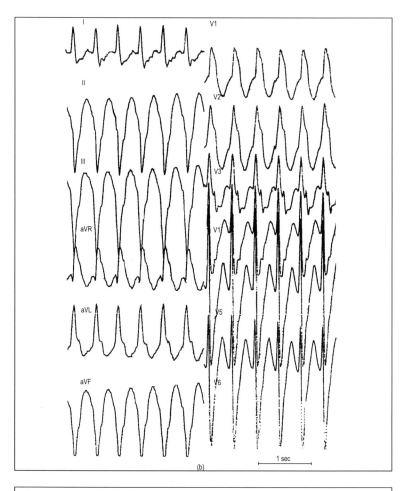

4(b) Ventricular tachycardia with right bundle branch block configuration

Notes on ventricular tachycardia (VT)

- regular rhythm @ 200 (+/-40) beats per minute
- broad qRS > 0.14 sec.
- the presence of p waves, capture beats or fusion beats favour the diagnosis. 40% of p waves may be retrograde.
- in V lead analysis, concordance (all qRS complexes positive or all negative) favours the diagnosis.
- the vast majority of such dysrhythmias in the context of ischaemic heart disease are VT.
- when in doubt, the management of a broad complex tachyarrhythmia as VT is likely to be effective and safe.

Appendix E

Coronary risk chart

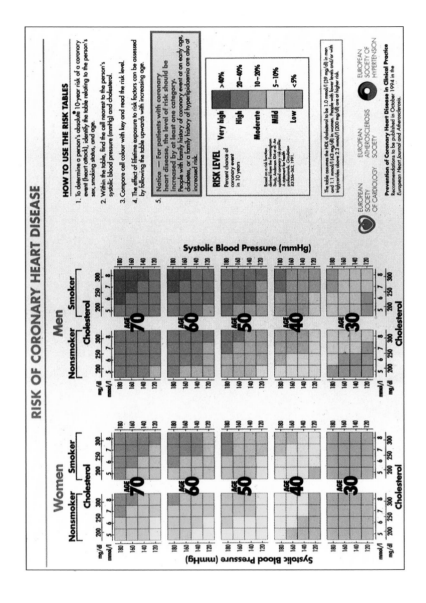

RISK OF CORONARY HEART DISEASE

HOW TO USE THE RISK TABLES

1. To determine a person's absolute 10-year risk of a coronary event (heart attack), identify the table relating to the person's sex, smoking status, and age.

2. Within the table, find the cell nearest to the person's systolic blood pressure (mmHg) and cholesterol.

3. Compare cell colour with key and read the risk level.

4. The effect of lifetime exposure to risk factors can be assessed by following the table upwards with increasing age.

5. Notice — For patients with coronary heart disease, the level of risk should be increased by at least one category. People with family history of coronary event of an early age, diabetes, or a family history of hyperlipidaemia are also at increased risk.

RISK LEVEL

Risk	Percent chance of coronary event in 10 years
Very high	>40%
High	20–40%
Moderate	10–20%
Mild	5–10%
Low	<5%

Based on a risk function derived from the Framingham Study, Anderson KM et al. An updated coronary risk profile. A statement for health professionals. Circulation 83:356–362, 1991.

The table assumes the HDL cholesterol to be 1.0 mmol/l (39 mg/dl) in men and 1.1 mmol/l (43 mg/dl) in women. People with lower levels and/or with triglycerides above 2.3 mmol/l (200 mg/dl) are at higher risk.

Prevention of Coronary Heart Disease in Clinical Practice. Recommendations to be published in October 1994 in the European Heart Journal and Atherosclerosis.

EUROPEAN SOCIETY OF CARDIOLOGY

EUROPEAN ATHEROSCLEROSIS SOCIETY

EUROPEAN SOCIETY OF HYPERTENSION

Lifestyles and Characteristics Associated with Increased Risk of Future Coronary Heart Disease

Lifestyles	General risk-factor advice	Biochemical or physiological characteristics (modifiable)	Personal characteristics (nonmodifiable)
Diet high in saturated fat, cholesterol, and calories		Elevated plasma total cholesterol (LDL cholesterol)	Age
Tobacco smoking		Elevated blood pressure	Sex
Excess alcohol consumption		Low plasma HDL cholesterol	Family history of CHD or other atherosclerotic vascular disease at early age (in man < 55 years, in women < 65 years)
Physical inactivity		Elevated plasma triglycerides	
		Hyperglycaemia/Diabetes	Personal history of CHD or other atherosclerotic vascular disease
		Obesity	
		Thrombogenic factors	

Priorities of Coronary Heart Disease Prevention in Clinical Practice

1 **Patients with established CHD** or other atherosclerotic vascular disease

2 **Asymptomatic subjects with particularly high risk** (subjects with severe hypercholesterolemia or other form of dyslipidaemia, diabetes, or hypertension; subjects with a cluster of several risk factors)

3 **Close relatives of**
   – patients with early-onset CHD or other atherosclerotic vascular disease
   – asymptomatic subjects with particularly high risk

4 **Other individuals met** in connection with ordinary clinical practice

Guide to Lipid Management

Total cardiovascular risk should be assessed first and the major components of risk identified. If 10-year CHD risk exceeds 20% or will exceed 20% if projected to age 60, **more intensive advice for all risk factors** will be required. **Clinical vascular disease** will increase the risk to more than 20% for most and to more than 40% for many.

Cholesterol level mg/dl	mmol/l	General risk-factor advice	Intensive physician- & dietician-led risk advice	Drug treatment considered if diet fails	Comment
350	9		YES	YES	Check fasting lipids. Exclude secondary hyperlipidaemias. Check family members
300	8		YES	YES if CHD risk >20%	Check fasting lipids. Exclude secondary hyperlipidaemia
250	7		YES if CHD risk >20%	Occasionally if very high risk	
200	6	YES	YES if CHD risk >20%		
	5	YES			

- Diet is the cornerstone of management.
- General risk-factor advice implies avoidance of tobacco, weight control, less than 30 percent of dietary calories as fat (of which less than a third are from saturated fat), control of hypertension, and frequent leisure exercise.
- Management decisions should not be based on a single cholesterol measurement. Laboratory variation may be 0.5 mmol/l (120 mg/dl) or more.

- Raised triglycerides signal the need for fasting lipid estimations (HDL cholesterol may be low). Hypertriglyceridaemia often responds to weight and alcohol control.
- The benefits or otherwise of drug treatment in women and in the elderly are unknown.

Guide to Blood Pressure Management

Total cardiovascular risk should be assessed first and the major components of risk identified. If 10-year CHD risk exceeds 20% or will exceed 20% if projected to age 60, **more intensive advice for all risk factors** will be required. **Clinical vascular disease** will increase the risk to more than 20% for most and to more than 40% for many.

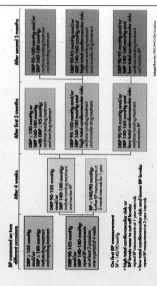

Appendix F

Useful references and suggested reading

ASPIRE Steering Group (1996) A British Cardiac Society survey of the potential for the secondary of coronary disease: ASPIRE (Action on Secondary Prevention through Intervention to Reduce Events) Principal results. *Heart*, **75**, 334–42.

Collins R., Peto R., Baigent C., *et al.* (1997) Aspirin, heparin and fibrinolytic therapy in suspected acute myocardial infarction *N Engl J Med*, **336**, 847–60.

Gibbons, R.J., Holmes, D.R., Reeder, G.S. *et al.* (1993) Immediate angioplasty compared with the administration of a thrombolytic agent followed by conservative treatment for myocardial infarction. *N Engl J Med*, **328**, 685–91.

Grines, C.L., Browne, K.F., Marco, J. *et al.* (1993) A comparison of immediate angioplasty with thrombolytic therapy for acute myocardial infarction. *N Engl J Med*, **328**, 673–9.

GUSTO (1993) An international randomized trial comparing four thrombolytic strategies for acute myocardial infarction. The GUSTO Investigators. *N Engl J Med*, **329**, 678–82.

ISIS-2 (Second International Study of Infarct Survival) Collaborative Group (1988). Randomized trial of intravenous streptokinase, oral aspirin, both, or neither among 17 187 cases of suspected acute myocardial infarction. *Lancet*, **2**, 349–60.

ISIS-4 (Fourth International Study of Infarct Survival) Collaborative Group (1995) A randomized factorial trial assessing early oral captopril, oral mononitrate, and intravenous magnesium sulphate in 58 050 patients with suspected acute myocardial infarction. *Lancet*, **345**, 669–84.

Julian, D.J., Braunwald, E. (eds) (1994) *Management of Acute Myocardial Infarction*. W.B. Saunders Company Ltd.

Kober, L., Torp-Pedersen, C., Carlsen, J.E. *et al.* (1995). A clinical trial of the angiotensin-converting-enzyme inhibitor trandolapril in patients with left ventricular dysfunction after myocardial infarction. *N Engl J Med*, **333**(25), 1670–6.

McGee, H.M., Browne, C., Horgan, J. Presentation and management of acute myocardial infarction in Irish hospitals. A national census (unpublished: manuscript in preparation).

Parisi A.F., Folland, E.D., Hartigan, P. (1992) A comparison of angioplasty with medical therapy in the treatment of single vessel coronary artery disease. *N Engl J Med*, **326**, 10–16.

RITA Trial Participants (1993) Coronary angioplasty versus coronary artery bypass surgery: the Randomized Intervention of Angina (RITA) trial. *Lancet*, **341**, 573–80.

Sacks, F. and the CARE investigators (1996) The effect of pravastatin on coronary events after myocardial infarction in patients with average cholesterol levels. *N Engl J Med*, **335**, 1001–9.

Scandinavian Simvastatin Survival Study Group (1994) Randomized trial of cholesterol lowering in 4444 patients with coronary heart disease: the Scandinavian Simvastatin Survival Study (4S). *Lancet*, **344**, 1383–9.

Swanton, R.H. (1994) *Pocket Consultant Cardiology*, Third Edition, Blackwell Scientific Publications.

Shepherd, J., Cobbe, S.M., Ford, I. *et al.* (1995) Prevention of coronary heart disease with pravastatin in men with hypercholesterolemia. The West of Scotland Coronary Prevention Study (WOSCOP). *N Engl J Med*, **333**, 1301–7.

Zijlstra, F., de Boer, M.J., Hoorntje, J.C.A. *et al.* (1993) A comparison of immediate coronary angioplasty with intravenous streptokinase in acute myocardial infarction. *N Engl J Med*, **328**, 680–4.

Index

Page numbers appearing in **bold** represent figures

Activated partial thromboplastin time
  (APTT) 14
Acute myocardial infarction
  Accident and Emergency
    Department care 11
  initial management 11
  presentation 1–10
  anterior 1, **2**
    Q-wave **3**
  anterolateral 1, **5**
  anteroseptal 1, **4**
  inferior 1, **6, 7, 9, 10**
  right ventricular 1
  true posterior 1, **8**
Acute pulmonary oedema 49–54
Adenosine 31, 48
  half-life 48
Adrenaline 54, 70
Advanced life support 80–2
Amiodarone 39, 43, 48
Angina 15
  unstable **17**, 25
  management 15, 19
Angiotensin converting enzyme
  inhibitors 29, 68
Anticoagulants 30, 68
Antitachycardia pacing 61
Aspirin 13, 29, 68
Atenolol 39
Atrial ectopics 31, **35**
Atrial fibrillation 39–43
Atrial flutter 39–43

Atrioventricular conduction
  defects 48–9
  bradycardias 49
  first degree AV block 48, **50**
  second degree AV block 49, **50, 51**
  third degree AV block 49, **52**
Atropine 31

Beta-antagonists (blockers) 21–2, 25,
  29, 39, 68
Broad complex tachycardia **46, 47, 48**

Calcium channel antagonists 25, 30
Cardiac arrest 79
Cardiac rehabilitation/secondary
  prevention 65–8
  driving 65–6
  exercise 66
  immediate measures 65
  mobilisation 66–7
  return to work 66
  sexual activity 66
  total risk evaluation 67
  total risk reduction 67–8
    diabetes 67–8
    hyperlipidaemia 67
    hypertension 67
    smoking 67
Cardiogenic shock 54
Cardiopulmonary resuscitation
  protocols 79–82
  basic 79–80

Chest pain 15, 19
Cholesterol 27
Complications of myocardial
  infarction 31–58
acute pulmonary oedema 53, 54
atrial ectopics 31, **35**
atrial fibrillation 39–43
atrial flutter 39–43
AV conduction defects, *see*
  Atrioventricular conduction
  defects
bradycardias 49
broad complex tachycardia 46, **47**,
  48
cardiogenic shock 54
sinus bradycardia 31, **33, 34**
sinus tachycardia 31, **32**
ventricular ectopics 43, **44**
ventricular fibrillation 43, **45**
ventricular tachycardia 43, **46**,
  47
Coronary angiography 19, 25, 64
Coronary care unit, myocardial
  infarction management 21–2
Coronary risk chart 92–3
Cyclimorph 21

DC shock 39, 43, 48
Deep vein thrombosis 57–8
Diabetes mellitus 67–8
Diamorphine 21
Digoxin 39
Diltiazem 30
Disopyramide 43, 48
Dobutamine 54, 71
Dopamine 54, 72, 73
  renal regimen 76
Dopexamine (Dopacard) 54, 74, 75
Dressler's syndrome 57

Echocardiography 63
Electrocardiogram (ECG) 63, 86–90
  exercise test 63

non-diagnostic changes with chest
  pain/unstable angina
  management 15–19
old inferior infarction **87**
pacemakers **88**
24–hour ambulatory
  monitoring 64
ventricular tachycardia **89**
  with right bundle branch
  block **90**
Esmolol 39

Follow-up treatment of post-
  myocardial infarction 29
Frusemide 53

Glyceryl trinitrate 21, 77
GTN spray 68

Haemodynamic monitoring 61–2
Heparin 25
Hypercholesterolaemia drug
  treatment 27
Hyperlipidaemia 67
Hypertension 67

Inferior myocardial infarction **6, 7, 9**,
  10
Intra-aortic balloon pump 54
Intracoronary stents 60
Isoprenaline 37, 69
Isosorbide dinitrate 21

Kussmaul's sign 23

Left bundle branch block **16**, 86, 89
Lignocaine 43, 48
Lipids, post-myocardial infarction
  management 27

Metoclopramide 21
Midazolam 48
Mitral incompetence, acute 55, **56**

Mobitz type 1 (Wenckebach phenomenon) 49, **50**
Mobitz type 2 49, 51
Morphine sulphate 21, 53

Naloxone 53
Nitrates 21, 25, 29–30, 68
Noradrenaline 54
Nuclear cardiology imaging 63

Overdrive pacing 48
Oxygen 21

Paroxysmal nodal supraventricular tachycardia **37**
Percutaneous transluminal coronary angioplasty 54, 59–60
Pericarditis 57
Posterior myocardial infarction, true **8**
Pulmonary embolism 57–8

Q-wave anterior infarction **3**

Right ventricular infarction 23–4

Sinus bradycardia 31, **33**, **34**
Sinus rhythm **36**
Sinus tachycardia 31, **32**
Smoking 67
Streptokinase 13–14, 69
Subendocardial myocardial infarction **17**, **18**

Tachycardia
  regular **36**, **37**
  supraventricular with right bundle branch block/aberrant conduction **38**
Temporary pacing 60–1, 83
Thrombolysis 11–15
  complications 14–15
    anaphylaxis 15
    bleeding 14–15
    hypotension 15
    reperfusion arrhythmias 15
  contraindications 13
  fast-track 12–13
  indications 13
  treatment protocol 13–14
Ticlopidine 60
t-PA 13, 14, 70

Unstable angina 25

Ventricular aneurysm, left 55, **57**
Ventricular ectopics 43, **44**
Ventricular fibrillation 43, **45**
Ventricular free wall rupture 55
Ventricular septal defect, acute 55, **56**
Ventricular tachycardia 43, **46**, **47**
Verapamil 39, 48, 69

Wenckebach phenomenon (Mobitz type 1) 49, **50**